Herbal & Nutritional Guide

DR. MARIE MICZAK

LOTUS
PRESS

P.O. Box 325
Twin Lakes, Wisconsin 53181

Disclaimer

This book is not a substitute for professional medical care and should be used with common sense and under the advice of your health care professional. The author and publisher are not responsible for use of the information in this book used outside of the scope for which it is intended, that being under your physician's supervision.

Copyright © 2004 Dr. Marie Miczak.
ALL RIGHTS RESERVED. No part of this book may be reproduced in any form or by any electronic or mechanical means including information storage and retrieval systems without permission in writing from the publisher, except by a reviewer who may quote brief passages in a review.

Cover & Page Layout & Design: Susan Tinkle

First Edition 2004
Printed in the United States of America

ISBN: 0-940985-68-3
Library of Congress Control Number:
   2003110455

Published by:
Lotus Press, P.O. Box 325, Twin Lakes, WI 53181 USA
web: www.lotuspress.com
email: lotuspress@lotuspress.com
800.824.6396

TABLE OF CONTENTS

DEDICATION

This book is dedicated to my daughter, Marie Anakee Miczak (the Hungarian Queen), who has contributed so much beauty to my life and work. Without her help, this book would have been nearly impossible. I love you so much more than words can ever express!

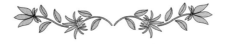

FOREWORD

Since time immemorial, the mystique, the aura, the shroud of misunderstanding has covered womankind. The essence of being a woman is in many cultures tied to superstition and folklore. Local tribal taboos exclude women from many facets of social life, specifically due to their menstrual flow. In fact, in some cultures of Africa and Latin America, women are precluded from being drummers or handling other musical instruments. This is because it is thought that her menstrual flow contaminates the purity of the music and its use in ceremonies. In other parts of Africa, primarily among the Islamic countries, women are still subjected to a mutilating form of disfigurement called female circumcision. Otherwise known as Female Genitalia Mutilation, or FGM, young girls between the ages of 5 and 8 are subjected to this barbaric practice, which often results in death due to subsequent infections. As the world becomes a more global community, excesses such as these are seen more and more often. They have always existed; however, due to isolation and lack of communication between countries and cultures, the secrets remained hidden to all but a few that have actually endured them.

We now have reporting by the World Health Organization that provides samplings of health-related issues affecting women all over the world. Not all atrocities against women are committed from within their own society. We have outside influences which, for-profit and gain, have exploited women and Third World countries. For example the multimillion-dollar company Nestlé had been marketing their infant formulas to impoverished women living in developing countries. The result was malnutrition and higher infant mortality rates due to the mother's inability to afford the formulas. This also caused an interruption in established breast feeding practices, which yielded heavier, healthier babies in the past. Mothers were given samples of the infant formulas without charge. After feeding the infants these products their own natural milk dried up. When they subsequently needed to purchase the infant formulas, they found that they had little money in the family budget to do so. The women, unable to afford this, began mixing inadequate amounts of the powders using contaminated water. This led to a serious problem with infant diarrhea, which to date is the biggest cause of young children's death in third World countries. So, here we see the womanly art of breast feeding has been undermined by corporate greed seeking to expand profits at the expense of both women's and children's health. Indeed it is a sad commentary.

Even in affluent countries, women are still not given access to the resources enjoyed by male members of the population. For example, there is still a distinct difference between what a woman is paid and what a man is paid to do the same job. The corporate glass ceiling is indeed a reality for many women who are accomplished in their field, are hard workers and who can contribute significantly to their company's success. Adding insult to injury, many times the same women are expected to do menial tasks in service to their male counterparts working in the same office. For example, who is it in your office that makes the coffee every morning? When there are special occasions or office parties, who generally makes the arrangements for refreshments for the guests? I think we all know the answer to these questions. It is almost a given that women are more "suited" for such activities. Most of us did not check off hospitality hostess on our job application when we first applied. How is it, then, that it becomes part of the job description once we are hired?

We can go on and on about the injustices that take their toll on both our health and psyche. Still, there is much more to be gained by focusing on what we can do for ourselves as women, drawing from the support of experiences spanning the eons. Let's face it, our foremothers survived despite quite difficult conditions. All of them contributed something that paved the way for us to be who we are today. Look back and you will see that this was no minor sacrifice. I think of my paternal grandmother, Jenny Hines, who worked in a Laundromat pressing shirts and suits. She enjoyed getting a perm at Bambergers department store and buying beautiful hats, gloves and shoes there as well. However, her family came first so in addition to her working outside of the home to help supplement her husband's paycheck, she worked equally as hard in the home. Her contributions to the family resulted in making my father an honest, hard-working, law-abiding citizen who himself took his family responsibilities quite seriously. That was her gift and her sacrifice to her family. At the age of 42 long hours in a hot, steamy Laundromat and equally long hours at home took their toll and she died as the result of double pneumonia. Look closely and you will see courageous women in your own family lineage that gave and loved you even before you were conceived. As women we think of the generations that will come from our womb, even though we may not live to see more than two or three. But it is this investment in the future that allows us to think beyond our own comforts of the day to provide a lasting foundation for our future progeny.

As you read through this book, I hope that you will see

that the choices you make today in caring for your own health almost certainly affect future generations. Just think of yourself as a pebble thrown into a pond. The concentric rings flow out from the impact you make. These are the generations coming after you. In caring for yourself, you set the standard of excellence of care for your daughters. Mothering is a learned profession. Children who are deprived of nurturing and attention, especially from their mothers, are impaired beyond measure. It is a stunting of the soul that is seen in a child who is not shown what love is. In this respect both my parents were exemplary. My mother taught me, "Nothing beats a failure but a try," which I value to this day. In this she showed me that she wasn't afraid to take a chance, whereas most women are taught to take a safe path instead. However, there is seldom any growth involved in following the beaten path. Had I not taken chances in life, I would not have experienced half of the joys of being human. Lessons that we teach ourselves flow over by example in teaching our children. By watching us, they witness the full potential for success available in themselves.

INTRODUCTION

How do I use this book?

This book is designed to take you through every phase of a woman's life cycle. In each phase you will find hands-on information and advice gleaned from years of case studies using real women just like ourselves. Each section explains health issues of importance to women in a way that dignifies the reader rather than make her feel that there's something inherently wrong with being female. Case in point, just look at commercials aimed at women. They indicate women need underarm deodorant, personal hygiene spray, super absorbent tampons; medication for before, during and after menstruation; and now a form of Prozac for PMS! The list is actually much longer, but I think you see my point. Beginning when we are old enough to understand a TV ad, we are bombarded with a message that it is not OK to be a woman. In fact it is a liability and the only thing that we can do to compensate for this mistake of nature is to purchase all of these products so that we can be "normal."

That is where this book comes in. Its intent is to liberate your mind from believing all of the media hype so that you can make truly rational decisions on issues that are of key importance to your health and well being. You see, in the flurry of all of this superficial foolishness, we forget what is the essence of vibrant health. Needless to say it does not come in a spray can. It also does not come in the latest shade of the season for lipstick at your local cosmetic counter. It is much deeper than that. It is caring for yourself and the confidence you exude as you present yourself to the world at your peak, both mentally and physically.

The best way to use this book is to chart where you are now and where you want to be in, let's say, five years. Age is not an issue! Five years from now, yes you will be five years older but if you work at it you will also be five-years smarter, stronger, healthier and more toned. We have no control over time but we do have control over our destinies. These variables are not age dependent. They are rather attainable by any one of us willing to reach out, make the commitment and follow-through.

Start with chapter two, which will begin to assess your starting point regardless of your age. You will also begin to see that much of how gracefully we age is more about choices we make right this minute as opposed to our gene pool. Each chapter that follows will help you to build upon what you have achieved in the previous chapter. Later on in the book, you can review the specific chapters that address your needs during specific phases of your reproductive cycle. These of course include your first menstrual cycle through menopause. The main point is that you are not a set of symptoms. You are a woman. That is why this information is placed in a separate section. You can pick and choose according to your current station in life the areas that apply to you.

The rest of the information is universal and can be applied during all phases of your reproductive cycle. This is what makes this book different from others on the subject. There is a difference between women's health and health for women, the latter being more expressive of a dedication to the improvement of the female gender rather than limping on complaints of being female. I think that we can all safely say that we have had enough of the latter.

As you read through this book, you may begin to take note of options available to you for future stages of your life. This would mean exploring alternatives to hormone replacement therapy while you are still menstruating. It is a known fact that as early as age 30 many women will begin to have a shift in estrogen production. While it is not noticeable at that age, the process has already begun. The average age of menopause for American women is somewhere around 52.7 years. However, you can be peri-menopausal for up to 10 years before your last cycle. Now that's a long time! You may notice symptoms long before the cessation of your cycles. During this time you may experience bone loss, sagging skin and thinning hair, which are things that you may not even attribute to the decrease in estrogen. We do not want to wait until that day is upon us to take action. Oftentimes a woman may be pressured into going on estrogen replacement therapy because her symptoms have become so unmanageable. I am referring to night sweats, hot flashes and vaginal dryness to name but a few. These are clear wake-up calls that estrogen is no longer being produced at the levels of your youth. This transition can be quite scary if one is not prepared. This is also where a woman may be more easily swayed to accept the standard medical treatment for menopause along with its assigned risks.

Hence, forewarned is forearmed. With the information found in this book, you will begin to understand what your body is going through at each stage and what you can do to maintain optimal health throughout. You need to keep an open mind and remember, plan for the future! How you take care of yourself today will have a huge impact on your menstrual cycles, your ability to conceive, your pregnancy, ease of childbirth and smooth transition into menopause. It's all in the planning.

Women's Health in Focus

Before discussing women's health concerns, keep in mind that most clinical trials for the testing of pharmaceuticals are done using male volunteers. Young females who may become pregnant are discouraged from participating due to the teratogenic effects that may be sustained by the fetus. A woman's hormonal make-up, body mass and weight make her needs especially unique as compared to men who tend to have more muscle mass.

Questions about the long-term effects of certain medications on the female population prompt concern now and for future generations. For example, Retin-A (trentinoin) was initially thought to be safe for use during pregnancy. After all, it is a derivative of vitamin A and is topically applied; in other words, it is a non-systemic drug. Currently there are precautions being discussed as this highly potent form of vitamin A may be absorbed enough through the skin to cause teratogenicity, or developmental defects, in unborn fetuses. More disturbing yet are the medications that can alter genetic codes, causing deformities for generations to come. These substances are known as mutagens and can be responsible for everything from birth defects to rare cancers. Not having time and experience on our side, we may well be playing Russian roulette with the human race.

It is very important for women to take control of their health by asking questions before blindly accepting the first medication protocol offered. Often times during our office visits we feel so pressured to not waste the doctor's time we accept a form of therapy we are not completely comfortable with. The doctor may not know all of the ramifications each drug may present and by the time you check with the pharmacist, you are picking up the filled prescription! At this point you are being informed after the fact, before you have had a chance to investigate all of the potential side effects and adverse reactions that may mean this type of drug therapy is not for you. Remember, most medication choices do not require a snap judgment and there is often time to consider other options or even a second opinion. This is your life! Don't be shy or think the doctor will consider you a difficult, hysterical patient. If he does, he is not attuned to your need for information or taking your healthcare very seriously, either.

The fact is, health consumers are becoming more educated and, as this book has demonstrated, looking for ways to *integrate* the best of orthodox and holistic medical approaches. Talk, read, study and listen until you are satisfied that you have been given access to all of the viable choices available to treat your specific condition.

An area of much misunderstanding is that of a woman's reproductive cycle. Shrouded in mystery from time's beginning, we see many taboos and rituals from all cultures surrounding the woman's menstrual flow, giving birth and menopause (sometimes called croning). Misconceptions by both men and women often make it difficult for the woman to enjoy the experience of each sexual stage of her life. Just look at how we associate these cycles with unpleasant terms. Which word more readily comes to mind?

Fill in the blanks:

1. Menstrual _____
    a) Flow
    b) Cramps
    c) Blood

2. Childbirth _____
    a) Joy
    b) Pain
    c) Energy

3. Menopause _____
    a) Dryness
    b) Freedom
    c) Phase

Well, if you are totally honest, more than likely you chose cramps to go with menstrual, pains to go with childbirth and dryness coupled with menopause! It is really not totally our fault, however. Just look at the commercials for products aimed at women. They practically make you think that being a member of the feminine gender is in and of itself a terminal condition. We are also twice as likely to self medicate than men, who will often "tough it out" or engage in some other activity until their symptoms dissipate. Actually, the "toughing it out" option is often better in many cases since over-medicating self-limiting illnesses is quite unnecessary.

In working to achieve our full potential for health and vibrancy, we must unshackle our minds from these negatives perpetuated by commercial interests that are only focused on selling us symptomatic relief. Stop and think why you may be having symptoms in the first place and *then* attack the underlying cause of the problem. Rather than give in to your discomforts, adopt a take no prisoner's attitude and obliterate them. Even so, you need to know specifically what you are dealing with.

Most symptoms we women suffer that are associated with our reproductive phases are due to the fluctuations of our delicate hormones. Estrogen, progesterone and even testosterone are all key players in how we feel emotionally and physically. It is when our hormones are out of balance that we begin to see such changes in our minds and bodies. A lack of understanding of this intricate dance can leave us thinking that there is something gravely wrong and we may opt for medical treatment that is inappropriate or even unnecessary. For example, did you know that doctors are now prescribing Prozac for PMS? Most depression associated with the menstrual cycle is transient so why would you want to be on antidepressant therapy 365 days of the year? Once again, this is an example of viewing the very essence of womanhood as a disease.

Over the past 20 years or so, methods of childbirth such as Bradley and Lamaze have defined a way to embrace and harness the energy of drugless parturition. These methods have actually empowered women to take an active part in birthing their babies. Birthing centers and home-birth options have also broken the traditional barriers of the 1940's and 50's whose protocols restrained and drugged women in order to control them during the ordeal of giving birth.

Another sign that we still have far to go in the area of liberated birth can be seen by the disproportionately high performance of cesarean sections here in the United States. Worldwide in other developed countries such as Great Britain we see roughly 11-15%. By contrast here in America our rate of C-sections comes in at about 33%, meaning that one in every three women giving birth will undergo a surgical procedure to do so.

This is shocking since Americans are known to be the most affluent, the most informed and the most advanced in medical care. Looking at statistics from *birthing centers* vs. hospitals throughout the country, you will find a clue. The number of women transported to birthing centers more closely resembles those of Great Britain, only even lower, between 5-10%. We have to ask how are our views of the normalcy of giving birth different in one setting over another? Is it that in a hospital we expect more medical intervention and procedures? Also, how much is done to avoid a malpractice lawsuit and how much is truly necessary for the patient's welfare? These may seem to be difficult queries but they are all one in the same. Taking part by discussing your needs with your health care practitioner will go a long way towards getting the care and attention both you and your baby deserve.

It is important to remember that hospitals have a bottom line. During the 1970's the warmth and home-like atmosphere of alternative birthing centers drew away potential hospital customers. In birthing centers caring, competent midwives attended women. The birth experience included their personal support system of husband, friends, parents and younger children in the family. In an effort to compete, hospitals began opening their own birthing rooms with pretty murals, soothing music and beds with wooden head boards just like home! The only thing is that you were still in a hospital, and even with all of this elaborate window dressing you still had a much higher risk of undergoing a cesarean section before you were done.

Finally I would like to briefly cover the next phase of the female reproductive cycle, menopause. All of our negativity regarding what it means to be a woman seems to pool here. For years we have complained about menstrual discomfort; however, now we take hormone replacement therapy so that we can have our menstrual cycle well into our 70's. There is obviously something wrong with this picture. When a woman enters menopause, the shifts in hormone production can be quite a lot to deal with. Hot flashes, vaginal dryness and other symptoms can make a woman feel old before her time. It is at such a low point that hormone replacement therapy, or HRT, may sound like the ideal solution. Given the fact that a woman's chance of developing breast cancer actually increases with age, you must consider that this risk is potentiated with prolonged exposure. This would also include the birth control pills you may have started taking in your 20's. This all adds up over time and as it has often been said, "estrogen is indeed the fodder of all female cancers." Indeed, we must take note of what is at stake here. It would seem that the media plays upon our worst fears of losing our health, our beauty and even our value as productive members of society, when none of this need be so.

The following chapters will provide a bit of insight as to what you can do now for yourself to avoid many of the symptoms so closely related to the female sexual cycle as well as conditions secondary to the natural decrease in estrogen. The key is to prepare now, wherever you are in the normal cycle of life, and begin to plan a strategy that is right for you alone.

Chapter 1

THE NEW MOON

Your First Menstrual Cycle

I f you are reading this chapter and think "This doesn't apply to me, I'm nearing menopause," please consider the following. All women are teachers. We are the first teachers to our children and oftentimes the first instructors to young people living in our community. Your impact cannot be calculated since there are so many young women in need of this information. For the sake of your daughters and all young women who come after, you need to read this chapter.

Many times parents would rather defer discussion of human sexual development to the school system. However, while your daughter may learn a bit about the mechanics of how her body works, nothing can replace personal experience and loving concern as provided by yourself. Armed with the information provided in this chapter, you will be able to employ a holistic approach to problems incidental to this phase of a woman's life. It is the human touch and involvement that makes this tedious transition so much easier for your daughter. I can remember my mother telling me that in my grandmother's day, it was not polite to discuss such things. My mother had no idea what was happening to her when she had her first menstrual cycle at age 12. She only recalls sitting at her desk in school and when she got up one of her classmates told her that she had "something" on the back of her dress. She ran to the rest room and saw a big stain of blood. She was so afraid that there was something wrong with her, not being able to discern the source of this bleeding. Later that evening, she confronted my grandmother about this. My grandmother told her that she was just too ashamed to discuss things like this with her.

Even today we may have reservations about speaking with our daughters concerning their changing bodies. Young women often get so much misinformation from their peers, which may well be due to the fact that they may not be getting any information at all from their mothers. My own mother's experience with her mother strengthened her resolve to teach me everything she knew before I even had my first menstrual flow. This was so appreciated because there were no horrific surprises. I can remember the date as being September 14th because it was my father's birthday! Rather than having a feeling of shame or dread, I can remember calling him at work and shouting my excitement that I had started having my periods. It was a milestone for me that I wanted to share but only because my mother had prepared me well for the day. The best advice is not to expect that someone else is going to do this job for you. There is no substitution for your personal experience in this area. Most likely, your daughter's menstrual symptoms will be very close to your own anyway. No book could anticipate that. So while you may be tempted to simply purchase a book for her on the subject, this will not imprint upon her your specific knowledge of your family's own makeup. You are very much necessary to her successfully coming-of-age.

The best thing you could do is to go through this chapter together. Consider yourself a tour guide pointing out all the areas of interest that would pertain to her own specific needs. Then you can see what aspects to focus on that will best help her. Since most young girls get the nuts and bolts of human sexual development in health class, we are not going to focus on that as much here. What we are seeking to do is provide complete support and information for this phase of a woman's life, which I call the new moon.

The term "New Moon" denotes growth. Cherokee farmers would often plant crops during the specific growth cycles of the moon. The "New Moon" is the phase of human growth that is a passing from childhood into puberty. Many changes will be seen prior to a young girl's first menstrual cycle. Still, many factors pursuant to when a young girl menarches are determined by heredity, diet and body weight. For example, it has been seen that American girls appear to be starting their menstrual cycles at least three to four years ahead of their European counterparts. Why is this? Well, many assume that this is due to the Superior American diet! However, it is seen that Americans are among the most overweight citizens of the world. What we are really seeing in our young people, especially girls, are children who are not getting enough exercise. Sitting in front of the computer and television accounts for a large percentage of many a young girl's recreational time. Also, fast foods have become more and more common additions to our diet. For example when I was a young girl there were very few, if any, restaurant chains. Oh yes, there were a few McDonald's franchises, but we seldom if ever went there after school. It just was not socially acceptable or desirable for young people to hang out at fast-food eateries at that time. Now the media makes it appear to be an accepted part of growing up!

With the higher caloric intake and less exercise to burn off these calories, our American girls are heavier and have a higher percentage of body fat to muscle by ratio than their European sisters. It is this extra body fat that facilitates the esterization of the female hormone estrogen. Puberty essentially begins when there is enough estrogen being produced by the body to initiate the first menstrual flow. This may be one of the reasons why European girls of a leaner build may begin their cycles a bit later. This can be borne out by the fact that American girls have consistently been reaching puberty at a younger and younger age since the turn-of-the-century, or the 1900's. Today, females in the United States generally will menarche between the age of 11 and 13. This is in stark contrast to young girls living in Europe who generally have their first cycle between the ages of 14 and 17. What ramifications does this have for long-term health? Primarily what is being seen is an increase in breast and uterine cancers in American women. The theory goes that the longer you are exposed to endogenous estrogen, or estrogen that is produced by the body, the greater your chances are for developing cancer. This correlation may be seen in women who had a delayed onset of puberty and exhibit less incidences of cancer later on in life. You may also choose to include many more variables in the mix, which I will address in this chapter. For example, another contributing factor is the American use of antiperspirants. Women who use such preparations may specifically be increasing their risk of developing breast cancer. This is due to the fact that the compound aluminum chlorhydrate physically blocks the pores, thus inhibiting the release of sweat. Included in our sweat are other compounds, toxins and impurities. With no avenue of natural release, the theory is that these products can sensitize breast tissue into cancerous mutations.

Our European counterparts consider being clinically clean a primary trait of American culture. In other words, we strive to have little or no natural human fragrance. In our quest to obtain this unrealistic goal we go to extreme methods, which in the long run will undermine our health and well being.

Another issue that you should discuss with your daughter is the correct type of bra to wear. Tight, constrictive bras impede the natural flow of lymph from the lymph nodes located in the areas of your armpits. In a similar fashion such attire acts like the antiperspirant. That having been said, it is very important to be fitted properly for your first bra and be measured regularly as your body changes. Not only will you have maximum comfort and freedom of movement, you may be insuring the future health of your breasts by doing so.

This is why this chapter is so important for both mothers and daughters. It lays the foundation for positive self-care and natural health choices that will last and benefit you throughout your life. Think of it as getting started on the right foot. If you are beyond this time period of your life, consider it a lesson in mentoring. As a mature woman you have so much to offer younger women who are so very much in need of this information. I encourage you to share it! By doing this we connect the circle of life by insuring that our younger sisters have every opportunity for health and well being. Try to remember the teacher or neighbor who gave you a leg up by providing you with some inside advice. Perhaps you were too embarrassed to ask your own mother about your menstrual cycle, birth control and pregnancy. Young women today need as much support as we can possibly give them. There are so many more complications to living now. Things that we did not even have to concern ourselves with 20 years ago are now commonplace realities of life. Date rape, abusive relationships and chemicals in our food and water increase the stress index, especially for young women. There is so much more anxiety and uncertainty about the future. Hence we must be signposts for our young sisters, giving them assurance and direction in a very frightening environment. We have to teach them that nice girls can say "no." We have to instill in them a sense of self-duty. We have to endow them with the tools they will need to survive.

Rather than give you a list of symptoms and remedies,

what I am trying to provide you with in this chapter is a healing of the whole person. The type of advice you give or accept will impress upon the young woman her valued place in the universe. We are so much more than just fluctuating hormones, cramps and water-weight-gain. We have to look beyond that and teach our young women that to properly care for yourself is a necessity for success in everything else that you do. We will therefore start with the basics and discuss issues dealing with a woman's first menstrual cycle, or menarche.

Your First Menstrual Cycle

This is such an exciting time for you! Your body is maturing and producing the appropriate hormones in just the right amounts to allow you to have your first menstrual cycle. With this new chapter in your life unfolding before your eyes, you are bound to have questions. In many cultures a mother or a female relative would talk to the young girl and instruct her on how to care for herself during her monthly flow. Among the Native American tribes of North America, specifically my own Iroquois, the tribal midwife or clan mother, who most often are one and the same, would teach you. Today, you may have already learned about this particular part of human anatomy in school. However the specifics on how to overcome common problems associated with your menstrual cycle were most likely lacking in this instruction. This is because there is a big difference between book learning and human interaction. Your mother or your aunt's own history may be a very telling factor in some of the patterns you yourself may form. For instance, perhaps your mother had her first cycle when she was 12, but often missed school due to severe cramps. This doesn't necessarily mean that this will be your lot, but oftentimes such sets of circumstances will run in families. That having been said, your first and foremost mentor should be your mother. If you have any doubt as to the importance of this informational link, just look at women who were orphaned. They will often go to great lengths to locate their biological mother just to ask her questions regarding their family health histories. If you are blessed to be living with your natural parents, please avail yourself of this valuable connection to your genetic past. Also, sharing this information will draw you closer to your mother. It shows that you truly value her opinion and insight enough to come to her at this critical turning point in your physical development. It also allows her to fully see what problems you may be having and to seek the appropriate help when needed. She is, after all, your mother and the person most intimately acquainted with your care since birth and interested in your welfare as you grow.

It is not my intention that you should make a chore out of mapping your menstrual cycle. However, there is an advantage to taking notes as to frequency, flow and symptoms associated with this time of the month. In my practice, I have had many young girls come to me with irregular cycles. Oftentimes the doctor would simply put them on birth control pills to establish a regular menstrual frequency. I consider this to be a very bad idea. Can you imagine a 14 year-old girl being prescribed birth control pills? In all reality I can't. This is because I know for a fact that prolonged exposure to estrogens over a lifetime will increase a woman's risk for developing breast and uterine cancer. Any such considerations of going on this form of hormonal regulation should be done with the utmost care. Sometimes it is just a matter of maturity or fat to muscle ratio that will cause the cycles to be irregular during the first year after menarche. Once established, and this may take a little time, you will find that there really is no need for such an aggressive solution. Patience is indeed the key.

My point is that before you jump ship and begin a form of hormonal regulation that you will most likely have to stick with indefinitely, a wait-and-see approach combined with a few natural food supplements and herbs may indeed prove to be the better solution. The beauty of such natural food choices is that they can be easily worked into the daily diet without much fuss or fanfare. Below is an example of how to do this using red raspberryherbal tea. It is absolutely delicious and nutritious and can help set a young woman's menstrual cycle right.

Red Raspberry Leaves *(Rubus Idaeus)* to Regulate Menstrual Flow and Ease Cramps

This was and still is a favorite plant of the Native American midwives of my tribe. The Latin-named *Rubus idaeus* species was cultivated in North America for thousands of years, having its roots in the earliest oral traditions of the Iroquois. As mentioned before, your tribal midwife or clan mother would help you learn the ways of womanhood. In such cultures, it was quite common for women to be isolated outside of the camp during their monthly flow. A small wigwam or dwelling was constructed just for this purpose. The midwives or medicine women would come and serve you during this time of isolation. Many women welcomed this time of the month because it was an opportunity to get away from the daily drudgery of chores. A woman could sew, cook or work on projects of interest to her during this time. Hence, every Native American woman was assured at least a monthly getaway!

As a menstrual tonic, red raspberry leaves have been used to quell the cramps and spasms associated with menstrual flow. Surges and ebbs of hormonal levels at the onset of a woman's cycle and corresponding dips in serum and red blood cell calcium as well as magnesium values can contribute to the muscle spasms and cramping that are so characteristic of menstrual discomfort. In an experimental study using 192 patients who were given magnesium daily for one week pre-menstrually and two days during the actual cycle, nervous tension was relieved in 89 percent of the participants. In addition, 96% experienced relief from breast pain and 95% noticed no apparent weight gain or bloating usually connected with their menstrual cycle.

One of the reasons why red raspberry leaves work so well for relieving all of the above symptoms is in fact due to the presence of organic magnesium and calcium. This form of magnesium and calcium is very easy to assimilate and absorb. Along with calcium and magnesium, Raspberry Leaves contain phosphorus, potassium and trace minerals, making it a complete mineral supplement in every way. As far as vitamin content, red raspberry leaves contain vitamin A, C, E and the B complex vitamins. You really can't get more complete than that! All of these factors along with the phytoestrogens present in the red raspberry leaves work to not only allay your discomfort, but help to normalize your cycle so that it is regular. Below is a basic recipe for a Raspberry leaf infusion that can be served either hot or cold.

Red Raspberry Leaf Tea

½ cup dried red raspberry leaves and berries

1 pint of freshly drawn water

Raw honey to taste (optional)

You may purchase red raspberry leaves in tea bag or bulk form from your local health food store. I personally prefer the bulk teas, which often include the berries in the mix. Delicious! If you choose the bulk form you will actually save money over purchasing the same amount in tea bags. However, you will need a metal tea ball or a teapot with a built-in strainer to steep the bulk herbs or tea bags. Steep one-half cup, or an ounce of the herb, in 1 pint of boiling water for 2 to 5 minutes. This is the standard infusion. It can be sweetened with raw honey to taste but I think you will find the sweetness of the raspberry fruits stand on their own. This herbal tea is rich in hormone balancing phytoestrogens and bioflavonoids, perfectly suited for problems associated with menstrual flow. One cup per day of this infusion is recommended for best results. The best part is that it is equally delicious hot or chilled. Therefore, in the summer when you may not feel like drinking hot tea, you can fix an iced tea version of this infusion for a refreshing cold drink on a hot day.

You can actually purchase or prepare your own tincture of red raspberry leaf rendered in either alcohol or glycerine. This can save you a bit of time since only a dropperful of this tincture added to a cup of hot water makes an instant tea. For complete instructions on how to make herbal preparations of all kinds, you might wish to refer to my book *Nature's Weeds, Native Medicine: Native American Herbal Secrets* also published by Lotus Press.

In any event, red raspberry leaf tea can be your first option when entering this phase of womanhood. While everyone is different, I have witnessed that most young women have normal cycles after taking this infusion for one month. As far as relief from menstrual cramps, backache and bloating, the results are seen in about a day. Keep in mind that at the onset of such symptoms, you may need to take two to three cups of the infusion to get more immediate relief. Hopefully you will see that this is not a Band-Aid® approach to these problems. What you are looking at is a tried and true herbal remedy that actually corrects the imbalances in hormonal production and mineral loss during this time of the month. Once your hormones are in balance and you are properly nourished, you will find a lessening or even an eradication of your symptoms altogether. This is the holistic approach, which employs the reasoning that a healthy body will function better and experience less discomforts.

To round out this regime, I would suggest taking a food based natural vitamin and mineral supplement with organic iron. Additionally, an easy to absorb calcium supplement in the amount of 1000 to 1200 mg per day should be added. Calcium is best absorbed when taken at night so you might wish to time the consumption of your calcium supplement with your dinner and just before bed. Try not to take any more than 500 mg at one time, though. This is because your body can only absorb approximately that amount at once. The wonderful thing about red raspberry leaves is that they are a food-based supplement. Many vitamins and minerals on the market today are coal tar derivatives. This means that they are not readily recognized by your body as food and are of limited value. Therefore a combination of the organic based nutrients found in the Red raspberry Leaves combined with a food based nutritional supplement is an excellent choice. If you are not tremendously fond of pills, you may wish to try nutritional powders. They can be mixed with water, milk or juice and immediately absorbed by the intestinal tract. The energy that you get from both the herbal infusions and the nutritional powders are superior to what you will find using any other supplements. If you still prefer to take vitamin and mineral pills, look for supplements that come in two piece gelatin capsules. These capsules release more readily in the digestive tract than their hard-compressed counterparts. If you doubt this, place a hard-pressed tablet and a gelatin capsule in a glass of room temperature vinegar. After 20 minutes look and see which form has broken down into aggregates. You will see that the gelatin capsule is the one that dissolves more readily, releasing its contents in the small intestines where it can do the most good. If your hard-pressed tablet is still in one piece, it is indicative of what is happening inside of you when you take it. That withstanding, using hard to digest products such as these is just a waste of your money.

PMS
New Findings, New Approaches

Carolyn DeMarco, M.D. addressed the causes and nutritional management of premenstrual syndrome (PMS), fibrocyctic breast disease and endometriosis. The most common aggravating factors include vitamin and mineral deficiencies and a diet high in sugar, meat, dairy and fat. Additionally dioxin, pesticides, chronic *Candida Albicans* (yeast infection), progesterone deficiency and emotional conflicts can intensify this condition.

PMS symptoms include, but are not limited to, breast swelling and tenderness, abdominal bloating and food cravings early in the menstrual cycle. Later in the cycle anxiety, irritability, breast pain, inward anger over aggressiveness and increased libido may be apparent. With 90% of all U.S. women polled having some PMS symptoms and approximately 10% having a severe form of this condition, practically every woman is affected.

Traditionally, medical treatment for PMS has been the prescribing of birth control pills until menopause. The next level of treatment has included tranquilizers, or even more drastically, the surgical removal of the hormone producing ovaries. Perhaps a more holistic approach would be to look at diet and lifestyle factors contributing to PMS. An estimated 15% of American women are deficient in iodine and mild hypothyroidism occurs in 90% of women with PMS. A correlation exists perhaps since our agricultural soils are often depleted of both iodine and chromium. The end result of low iodine/chromium food crops is obvious here. Supplementation can begin to bridge the gap in these deficiencies.

Following is a suggested list of nutritional supplements, along with dosages, to use for PMS:

Menstruating Women's Nutritional Protocol

(Complete formulas and preparation instructions can be found in *Nature's Weeds, Native Medicine*, Lotus Press)

Iron Tonic

A good source of absorbable, non-constipating organic iron.

¼ cup dried yellow dock root

¼ cup dried rose hips

¼ cup dried dandelion root

¼ cup dried alfalfa

This formula is very safe and effective in bringing up the hematocrit in iron deficiency anemia. This blend can be taken as a tea or finely ground and put into gelatin capsules.

Menstruating Woman's Blend

½ cup dried red raspberry leaves and berries

1 tsp. powdered wild yam root

¼ cup dried red clover blossoms

¼ cup dried chamomile

The rich amounts of magnesium, calcium and B-complex vitamins found in this blend help to quell PMS symptoms before they start.

Additional Daily Supplementation

400 IU vitamin E

200 mg chasteberry extract (during the second two weeks of your cycle beginning on day 14 with day 1 being the first day of your period).

1,000 –1,500 mg of calcium (the best source is microcrystalline apatite and the second is calcium citrate).

Aromatherapy for Menstrual Discomfort

Another option that you may wish to explore is the wonderful world of aromatherapy. I have taught aromatherapy at Brookdale College in Lincroft, New Jersey for many years. This course has evolved from a basic lecture to a workshop that allows the students to make and blend their own aromatherapy products. I have now expanded this course to a daylong spa that allows the students to fully experiment with and enjoy the benefits of essential oils for an entire retreat. The focus here is not so much on what we take internally. If you have an aversion to taking herbal teas or swallowing pills and nutritional powders, then this may be the perfect option for you.

Aromatherapy is the science of olfactory stimulation of the endocrine system via inhalation of plant essences. Simply put, employing the inhalation of the plant molecules into your system. These plant essences, or essential oils, are steam distilled and often use several hundred pounds of plant material. These essential oils are highly potent and concentrated; therefore, only a small amount is needed. The variety of ways to enjoy and utilize essential oils is as diverse as your imagination. Diffusers, lamps, sachets or in the bath, the list is nearly endless. What is even better is the fact that you can receive almost immediate relief from menstrual tension and cramps by taking a warm bath in an essential oil specific for this time of the month. You could even use essential oils to help regulate your hormones during the month so that when your cycle comes around, most likely you will have no symptoms at all. Remember, it is the fluctuation and imbalance of female hormones that causes the majority of the problems in the first place. Your goal should be to achieve the normalization of your hormonal output so that you ease into your monthly flow without any pain or discomfort. Aromatherapy really makes this easy because, as I mentioned previously, there are so many applications and ways to add their benefits to your daily life. The following formula is a form of diffusion that incorporates the use of warm water as a conduit for the essential oils. You could even use the same mixture in a hot tub (Jacuzzi®), sauna or steam bath. It is the heat and vapor that carry the essential oils to the limbic system, or our "smell brain," which is directly wired to the outside environment. Therefore, what you smell does not need to go through specific processing centers of the brain. Instead, the molecules of the essential oils go directly to the rhinencephalon portion of the brain where the molecular compounds stimulate the production of natural hormones within the body. This allows for quick and complete relief of menstrual symptoms. What is best is that these particular bath oils require no special equipment to use. No expensive diffusers, lamps or gadgets are necessary. All you need is a bathtub full of warm water and the essential oils themselves:

Clary Sage & Rose Bath Oil

   5 drops clary sage essential oil (*Salvia sclarea*)
   3 drops rose essential oil (*Rosa centifolia, Rosa dama-scena*)

It just doesn't get any easier than this! Draw your usual bath water making sure it is nice and warm. Just before climbing in add five drops of the pure essential oil of clary sage and three drops of the rose oil. As soon as the essential oils meet with the warm bath water they begin to vaporize into the air. This method of using aromatherapy is called diffusion. The molecules of the essential oils diffuse into the air and surround your bath. Also, any residual amounts of the essential oils left in the bathtub will diffuse through the many layers of your skin. The clary sage is a quick and sure regulator of female hormones. Clary sage is a muscle relaxant, it relieves stress and tension and addresses menstrual irregularities and cramps. You might even wish to use it prior to your menstrual cycle. The rose oil has anti-depressant qualities and also helps regulate the menstrual cycle. What exists in this formula is what is called a synergy. The two essential oils combined are far more powerful than if you were to use them separately!

Following is another formula that will also provide relief from menstrual discomfort while regulating your cycle to a normal rhythm:

Jasmine & Fennel Bath Oil

> 5 drops jasmine essential oil (*Jasminium grandiflorum*)
>
> 5 drops fennel essential oil (*Foeniculum vulgare*)

Similar to the previous formula, this blend will also help to stimulate the normal production of female hormones so that your cycles are normal and regular. The jasmine is a very exotic essential oil. Extracted from the jasmine flower, it is a wonderful complement to the female persona. It has strong anti-depressant qualities and is excellent in relieving menstrual pain and its associated cramps. Fennel is also excellent for premenstrual symptoms since it also helps to regulate the menstrual cycle. It is recommended that you try both of these formulas to see which one you prefer since we all have our own personal likes and dislikes. You might just fancy the clary sage-rose blend over the jasmine and fennel or vice versa, so it is good to have a few selections to choose from. Also, when you purchase essential oils you will find that the prices will vary. Depending on availability and your pocketbook you may choose essential oils that are less expensive but just as effective. Including essential oils as part of your daily bathing and body care routine is a very easy way to benefit from their properties. How often do we forget to take our vitamins or food supplements? However, even on our most forgetful of days we will not forget to bathe!

You may be tempted to try some of the commercial body washes that tout the inclusion of pure aromatherapy oils. I would pass them up if I were you. This is because many companies will use the cheaper fragrance oils that are chemically manufactured instead of the naturally-derived plant essential oils. While a product may smell lovely, it does not have the complex and beneficial essential oils with all their inherent properties and usefulness. Most importantly, your body will not be fooled by these phony fragrances! My advice is to purchase the pure, steam-distilled natural essential oils and add them to your bath as I have instructed. In the long run you will save both your money and your health by using a whole and natural product that has been tested over time. Additionally, you will have much greater versatility when using pure essential oils as opposed to products that only claim they contain them. You can take those same plant essences and make your own massage oil, body lotion, and shampoos. Once you have purchased the genuine article, they can be added to a variety of carriers for whatever purposes you wish. For more information on the Internet regarding the benefits of aromatherapy visit Suite101.com's special section at www.suite101.com/welcome.cfm/aromatherapy where you will find excellent articles and information about this fascinating science. You may also want to visit my Web site at www.miczak.com. In addition to information on aromatherapy we have links to various sites concerning the benefits of aromatherapy as well as book reviews and articles.

SUMMARY:

I hope that what I have presented here demonstrates that every stage of a woman's life is exciting and challenging. Rather than dreading coming-of-age, you should rejoice in the fact that your body is developing as nature has planned. Knowledge replaces fear and wisdom replaces ignorance. It is time to let go of age-old taboos and negative thoughts associated with our monthly flow. There is so much that we need to overcome by way of preconceived notions regarding our femininity. For example, while we all need to choose what type of feminine protection is best for us, we needn't buy into the media hype that we should purchase every deodorant and feminine hygiene spray available on the market. There are also options and alternatives to tampons and sanitary pads that you may not even know about. To give you an idea, there are natural tampons available that are made of green cotton and other natural materials. If you have ever wondered what women used before the advent of disposable sanitary napkins, look at the natural materials available to women at the time. At the turn-of-the-century women would tear old cotton sheets that were worn and softened with time and fashion them into pads for use during their cycle. Today you can buy pure cotton sanitary pads from specialty stores that specifically cater to women. Some are made out of green cotton, a term for cotton that has not been processed or bleached. It is actually beige in color, the true natural hue of cotton. In any event, green cotton products are a refreshing natural alternative to use in place of the chemically processed materials currently on the market.

Likewise, we must overcome age-old ideas as to what causes menstrual cramps and discomfort. I can remember my mother saying that cramps were caused by walking around barefoot before your cycle. She also said not to get your feet wet, which in and of itself is not a bad idea, but it does very little for aches and pains during your period. Most women still rely on over-the-counter preparations that are supposed to deal with a variety of premenstrual symptoms such as bloating, headache and cramping. Many of them contain basic components such as aspirin and caffeine. The aspirin is a common anti-inflammatory and analgesic, or pain reliever. The caffeine actually speeds up the effectiveness of the aspirin but it is also a mild diuretic. Therefore, the caffeine component is what helps relieve the excess water weight gain. While such preparations are not bad per se, they can only offer relief of the symptoms, not of the underlying causes of your menstrual distress. As previously outlined, the addition of absorbable calcium and magnesium are going to do far more for you than any drugstore preparation.

This is because your body needs these nutrients. When they are lacking is when we experience such problems. We have yet to establish the human body's need for aspirin and caffeine, however. What this should tell us is that balancing our nutritional requirements and utilizing supplements that the body easily recognizes as food is indeed our best defense. We should be more concerned with nourishing rather than medicating as the latter has limited long-term benefits, if any. Added to this dilemma are the other ingredients that are common to many over the counter menstrual relief products. Read the label and you will see added dyes, excipients, binders, waxes, fillers, etc. You will need to ask yourself what value these items have in contributing to your overall health and well being? It is my hope that if you follow through on the suggestions in this chapter, you will build optimum health and not require any of these medications to deal with that difficult time of the month. I have used every product that I have recommended in this section with resounding success. I can honestly say that I have been symptom free for years as regards my monthly cycle, which is more regular than most calendars!

Recently we are seeing a continuing rush to overmedicate. Now that pharmaceutical companies can directly market their drugs to consumers, you will see what I consider a rash of commercials aimed at women undergoing difficulties related to their menstrual cycle. This medication is actually a form of Prozac! The commercials show women out of control, irritable and weepy, all supposedly due to a new form of premenstrual disorder. The fact is that very few women actually have a clinically defined form of premenstrual syndrome. However, these commercials never indicate this and allow women to feel that this problem is far more widespread than it is. Hence, we have the solution in pill form. Since this newly prescribed medication is, once again, a form of Prozac, it actually can only deal with the depression and mood swings present during premenstrual stress. Prozac works by regulating the serotonin levels in the brain, not by balancing the more delicate female hormones. At best you are only dealing with a small portion of the total problem. Also, what does this say about women? Well, it is telling our younger women that there may be something inherently wrong with being female. That we are so inadequately made, medication is required at every turn, even for something as natural as our monthly cycle. This is perhaps the greatest insult of all. In the new commercials you witness women acting as if they need to be institutionalized, let alone medicated! Screaming, fits of anger, unable to remove a shopping cart from the rack; all of this supposedly due to your menstrual cycle. Unbelievable.

This also opens the door for a broad labeling of any woman who from time to time asserts herself and, yes, even gets angry. Is every woman who voices her opinion or takes an unpopular stand then said to have this disorder? If that is the case, what medication is given to middle-aged men, let's say in their 50's, who account for most of the violent incidences of "road rage?" The answer as you know is none. If you think about it, anger behind the wheel of a potentially deadly weapon has far more dangerous repercussions than a woman who verbally vents her frustrations. Armed with this new diagnosis aimed at controlling women's behavior and actions, she may be pressed into taking a medication that she really doesn't want or need. The commercials say it all. One moment the woman is an absolute wreck. She can't find her keys, she can't speak to anyone without exploding and to make matters worse her pants don't fit! We need to be so careful that we do not buy into this media hype. While many medications are indeed a lifesaver, a proper diagnosis should be obtained before taking this and any another prescription medication.

We have to learn to trust ourselves as well. It is so easy to buy into what commercials indicate true femininity and womanhood should be. Look at all the things we are expected to do. Shave our bikini line, underarms and legs. Cover our own natural scent with perfume and deodorant. Obsess over not being ultra thin. The list is too long to cover here, but for our purposes you can consider the following. Begin accepting yourself for the unique woman that you have become. This begins with accepting your positive attributes and gifts.

Oftentimes, low self-esteem begins with comparing ourselves to others. This is very dangerous, as even those who we admire the most have flaws and problems that we may not see. We imagine that the grass is always greener on the other side and that everyone else's life is truly sublime. This is not always our fault. Celebrities, movie stars and media people are exalted to almost a demigod status in our society. It seems no matter what they do, they are always "marvelous" and intriguing people. The truth, if allowed to be told, is that many of them are complete failures in both their personal and family lives. Multiple marriages, infidelities and drug and alcohol abuse abound. I do not think I need to go on. The tabloids have a field day and the players give them their money's worth. But at what price? Our young women are equating success with self-exploitation. Our daughters are learning that the world rewards behavior that borders on exhibitionism. Our next generation of women is being fed the lie that pleasing men is what counts in life. Self-respect takes a back seat to self-promotion. Yet when the smoke clears, we will eventually age, and these values we have embraced will no longer serve us. You see, if you have not made an investment in the sum and substance of who you are as a woman early on, you are surely headed for spiritual bankruptcy later on in life. If you are so focused on your looks and beauty, when they fade, what then will you have to offer? This is where many women hit rock bottom. You have seen them. Women who are in their 50's and 60's who still haven't a clue as to who they are as people. They go to the same bars and haunts, flirting as if they were still 18. The sad issue is that in all of these years they have yet to find an enduring relationship to which they can give and be given to. Time has passed them by. They still dress and act as if they are stuck in a time warp, totally out of step with today's pace.

The foundation that we have laid here is a tool for teaching and passing on wisdom to our younger sisters. Once again, the best way to achieve this is by setting the most positive examples and willingly sharing them with the world.

Chapter 2

THE HALF MOON

Your Childbearing Years

I f you have taken the time to read through Chapter 1, you will see that the focus is on enhancing your femininity, not correcting it. Thus, this philosophy should follow into your childbearing years to serve you well. Likewise, the foundation of proper self-care, nutrition and the judicious use of herbal preparations will prepare you for this phase of your life.

The reason I began teaching younger women how to care for themselves is because what they do as teenagers will have a major impact on their reproductive health as they mature. Oftentimes we think that as long as we eat well and do not smoke or use drugs during pregnancy, all the sins of the past are quickly forgiven. This is perhaps the greatest fallacy of all. You cannot just suddenly become a healthy person during your pregnancy. It takes years and years of proper nourishment and care. This may well account for an increasing number of women who are turning to fertility clinics in order to conceive. Problems commonly found during the teenage years such as anorexia and bulimia only show their true damage later in life. Similarly, over-consumption of junk foods and abuse of alcohol and drugs will impact greatly upon a woman's future health. The best advice of course is to never start with these self-destructive habits in the first place. However the reality of the situation is that when we are young, we feel that we are truly invincible. We may skip meals and not feel the worse for it. Perhaps we may have even smoked, but it didn't really slow us down or keep us from being on the girls' basketball team. This is because our bodies in our youth are quite forgiving. Still while our bodies may be forgiving, they certainly do not forget the abuse we have heaped upon it. They show up later on in life as deficiencies and abnormalities of growth, which can affect our ability to conceive and carry a pregnancy to term.

Even if your teenage years were less than perfect, you can still improve your health and well being now. Preparation for pregnancy is something that all young women who are contemplating marriage should consider. The time to make the positive changes that will best affect the future health of your children is during your early 20's. This means getting an adequate amount of calcium and folic acid, especially. While I am not narrowing down your nutritional needs to just these two supplements, they are mentioned because of their importance during the childbearing years. A full array of natural, food-based nutrients is indeed important. Still, you may have to give special attention to these nutrients due to the fact that many young women do not receive adequate intake of them. Take calcium, for example.

You may not know that most of the cheaper calcium supplements are made from calcium carbonate, which is derived from rock! Hardly anything your body could ever hope to absorb. Rather than becoming part of the natural bone matrix, calcium carbonate primarily gets stored in the soft tissues and can cause kidney stones over time. This is not what we take calcium supplements for. In your list of recommended nutritional supplements for the childbearing years you will find that the type of calcium I recommend is highly absorbable. It is actually made from natural bone and contains all of the macro and trace minerals necessary to replenish normal bone density.

As for the matter of folic acid, there was clinical evidence available as early as 1977 that this nutrient plays an important role in preventing neural tube defects. When I was pregnant with my second child, my midwife recommended that I take extra folic acid over and above what was provided in my prenatal supplement. At that time most pregnancy vitamins only contained about 400 mg of folic acid or less. Studies indicated that the amount recommended to help prevent birth defects was indeed much higher, actually around 800 mg per day. Even with this knowledge as provided by clear clinical assays, pharmaceutical companies were reluctant to add the appropriate amount of folic acid to their prenatal supplements. Why? The reason given was that higher levels of folic acid present in the body masks pernicious anemia. This condition, however, primarily effects 40 to 80 year-old patients, hardly the segment of the population that is likely to be pregnant! Therefore, because there was a potential of masking a disease that affects a small percentage of the population who are not likely to be pregnant anyway, this important nutrient was not supplied in the necessary amounts. In 1983 my midwife was very knowledgeable regarding the importance of nutrition for expecting mothers. She recommended that I take at least 800 mg of folic acid during my pregnancy. There are currently several studies linking folic acid deficiencies to not only neural tube defects but also low birth weight for gestation or age, which would indicate the key role folic acid plays in fetal growth. Adequate nutrition is not only important to help prevent neural tube defects such as spina bifida, but it may influence your ability to conceive in the first place. This is why preparation for pregnancy should begin long before you even contemplate conceiving.

Healthy Conception &
a Full-term Pregnancy

These two objectives may appear to be separate but they are actually interrelated. Many women today are experiencing great difficulty conceiving for the first time. Perhaps this may be due to women waiting until they have established their careers before starting a family. There are many factors to consider that may account for this trend; namely the fact that most of us today are not willing to wait very long for anything. The added pressure of the biological clock ticking away as you near the end of your reproductive cycle is a major catalyst.

Generally you can begin to suspect an infertility problem if, after one year of not using contraceptives, you do not conceive. Many women give up much sooner than that and begin taking medical measures to correct what they may perceive as an infertility problem. The solution is often expensive, time-consuming and even more stressful than the infertility itself. It also places pressure on both marriage partners as one ultimately blames the other for not being able to have children. For a man, his pride and masculinity are intertwined. Even suspecting that he could be the cause of the couple's infertility is a striking blow. For a woman, her confidence in her femininity is often related to her ability to do what the rest of womankind can do.

Giving birth is as natural an aspiration for many women as is a normal need to love and be loved. Babies and children provide this unconditionally. Just think about having your worst hair day and feeling totally unattractive to the outside world. Do you think your infant minds? Absolutely not. She may love you all the more for it. Parent/child relationships are much more enduring than marital relationships. You can have an ex-husband, but who ever heard of having an ex-child? Hence the need and desire to have children is strong and natural.

There are things that you can and should do in preparation. First of all you should make sure that you have enough folic acid by consuming 800 mg per day at least three months prior to your plans to conceive. You see, it is the early stages of fetal development that are so sensitive to deficiencies in this nutrient. Without adequate folic acid, the spinal column's outer sheath may not form properly. The effects of neural tube defects such as spina bifida are lifelong and in many cases debilitating. Your baby is especially vulnerable during the first three months when you may not even be aware that you are pregnant. In anticipation of pregnancy, get into the habit of not drinking alcohol, coffee or caffeine-containing drinks such as cocoa and cola drinks. Also avoid aspirin and antacids. Prior to conception observe that environmental risks including second-hand cigarette smoke, radiation from x-rays, cat feces, pesticides and paint thinners or solvents are avoided. Once you are pregnant, steer clear of prolonged exposure to extremely high temperatures such as those found in hot tubs, whirlpools and saunas.

While low impact aerobic exercise may be fine for non-pregnant women, it is not well suited for expecting mothers. This is due to the theory that during high peaks in the exercise activity, you may actually be depriving the baby of needed oxygen.

I think the best thing that you can achieve is a happy medium where you are aware of the possibility that during your childbearing years you could potentially conceive at anytime. That is why I took precautions and made decisions during this time of my life that served me well. One such case occurred when I was in my mid-30's and sought help for my adult acne. Dermatologists suggested that I go on Accutane®, a highly potent vitamin A derivative. One of the known side effects of using this drug was that it caused teratogenesis. This means that if I conceived while taking this medication there was an extremely high chance that my baby would be born deformed. In order to prevent a subsequent lawsuit as a result of this, the doctor insisted that I sign an agreement stating that should I conceive while taking Accutane®, I would have an abortion! This was totally unreasonable and I refused to take the medication or sign any such consent form. Medications such as these are stored long term in your liver. So, even after you stop taking it, there may be enough left in your system to cause damage many months after discontinuance. Do you want to take that risk with your child's future health? For me it just wasn't worth it and I have never looked back with regret.

The plant kingdom provides a wide variety of nourishing preconception and pregnancy botanicals. The first botanical I introduced was red raspberry leaves, or *Rubus species*. In addition to being a wonderful menstrual cycle regulator, its benefits extend into conception. When you have an irregular menstrual cycle, let's say you get your period every two months or even less, this is an indicator that your hormone production is inadequate. If you are producing the correct amounts of estrogen and progesterone, your cycle should come about every 28 days or so. This is an average cycle and indicates a healthy environment for conception. Native American midwives saw the value of red raspberry leaf. They recommended its use prior to conception and for women who are prone to spontaneous abortion or miscarriage. Clinical study indicates that the raspberry plant has been shown to be appreciably high in easily absorbable calcium and magnesium. Quite interestingly, these are the two minerals considered to be essential in effecting a woman's ability to become pregnant and circumvent premature labor and delivery.

Taken during pregnancy and in preparation for labor and childbirth, many women have found red raspberry leaves to be truly indispensable. Its reputation as a uterine toner is well founded. According to Dr. S. Kurzepa, a prominent biochemist, "Raspberry leaf tempers the effects of hormonal runaway such as might occur during menstruation, pregnancy and delivery." As a uterine muscle tonic, raspberry leaf helps facilitate parturition, or delivery, by normalizing the tone of the specific muscles involved. Many women have reported an easier labor and delivery with use of this time-honored plant. For the postpartum period, raspberry leaves combined with other nourishing herbs such as alfalfa, nettles, and blessed thistle encourage a copious supply of high-quality breast milk. These herbs also help to restore depleted energy and nutrient levels in the mother. In addition, herbal teas can help to provide the proper hydration that prepares the new mother for the fluid volume demands of lactation.

Recommended Pre-pregnancy Supplements

- Natural, food-based vitamin and mineral supplement
- Folic acid 800 mg
- Calcium in the form of microcrystalline apatite 1,000 – 1, 200 mg per day
- Magnesium

or

- Prenatal vitamin and mineral supplement with at least 800 mg of folic acid added
- Calcium in the form of microcrystalline apatite 1,000 – 1,200 mg per day
- Magnesium

Most commercial nutritional supplements on the market today are coal tar derivatives. These are synthetic vitamins that your body cannot recognize as a source of food and energy. You would do much better to use food-based nutritional powders or, if you prefer, supplements that are encapsulated in gelatin. Another option is to simply take a prenatal vitamin and mineral supplement prior to conception. This is quite a brilliant idea as you will be getting the appropriate amount of folic acid along with other nutrients crucial to nurturing a growing fetus. The new generation of food-based nutritional supplements for pregnancy is much easier to digest than the prescription vitamins of years ago. I can remember taking huge pink-colored horse pills called Natilin. They often repeated on me and made the morning sickness that I had all day even worse. This was over 20 years ago and that is what the doctor prescribed, so that is what I took. Most certainly it was better than nothing, but I have to wonder what benefit the artificial coloring and flavoring had in common with holistic nutrition.

The recommended supplements are considered the bare bones of your nutritional outline for conception. The trick is to keep it simple so that compliance is achievable. If you start loading yourself down with too many pills, you will find yourself not taking them at all. Whichever program you choose, you can get the most out of your dietary supplements by taking them with food. Nutritional supplements are better absorbed in the presence of other complementary vitamins and trace minerals. Not only that, your vitamins and minerals can cleave onto a protein molecule consumed during your meal and be easily assimilated in the small intestine. Another option to increase absorption and bioavailability is to make sure that any minerals included in your nutritional supplement are chelated. This is a chemical term used to describe combining a mineral with a ring structure. The end result is a "holding onto" the metallic ion much as a claw would grasp an object. In simple terms, that allows the body to utilize macro and trace minerals to their fullest potential.

Herbs for Fertility

You may also be interested in learning which herbs have been traditionally and safely used to increase fertility. Old wives' tales abound in this category! However, we are concerned with what is safe and efficacious. Keep in mind what was previously addressed in Chapter 1. Remember, one of the main goals is to regulate the delicate balance of female hormones so that the menstrual flow will cycle itself to about every 28 days. If you are cycling much less than that, let's say every 60 days, then you are only affording yourself half as many opportunities to become pregnant. Ovulation correspondingly occurs every 60 days as well if this is your normal cycle. Do you see how your chances to conceive are actually cut in half?

Regulation is the key. As previously addressed, the red raspberry leaf is ideal in achieving this purpose. Not only that, very few herbs can match it for its richness in vitamins and minerals. When menstrual regulation and optimal nutrition are combined they make for a powerful force towards your goal of becoming pregnant. Rather than taking multiple herbal teas and products during this crucial time, I would suggest these two very safe and time-honored herbs for both a nutritional boost and preparing the most receptive environment for childbearing:

Herbal Fertility Blend

¾ ounce red raspberry leaves with fruits

¼ ounce red clover leaf with flowers

This blend can be brewed as per the directions for most infusions. That would be 1oz total herbal tea blend to 1 part freshly drawn boiling water. If you choose the loose or bulk tea, which is usually more economical, you will find that packing your herbs into a tea ball before steeping is perhaps the best method. Steep the tea for 3 to 5 minutes or a little longer if you prefer a stronger brew. This particular blend is delicious with or without honey. It can be served hot or iced and taken in the amount of about one-half cup per day if you are preparing for a pregnancy. This is a very simple brew that is so very refreshing and good tasting. You will find yourself enjoying the journey to conception!

Breastfeeding Success

The best start for your baby begins at the breast. Despite all of the controversy over the past 25 years, nothing else has been found to match breast-feeding for the immune factors and superior nutrition breast milk offers. Unique to breast milk is the high content of "brain fat" it contains. This type of fat is necessary for optimal brain growth and development in the infant. It is suspected that it is the presence of this kind of fat that accounts for the higher IQ's associated with children who were breast-fed as babies.

Extending this experience may be of even more benefit. For example, in most parts of the world children are breast-fed well into toddler-hood and usually weaned by age three or four. This gives the child the best start and continued immunity throughout that time. It also supplies the much-needed brain fat that may be difficult to obtain through the local diet. These children are often calmer, more secure and adjust better to new and stressful experiences. The brain fat present in the milk may also have a beneficial effect on the entire central nervous system, allowing it to develop normally in the child. Our timetable for weaning often goes by what we think our neighbors or family will say and this is wrong. Listen to what your *baby* has to say. He or she may need that extra warmth and cuddling at the end of a busy day. This is a rare opportunity to re-bond with your toddler, especially after you have been away all or part of the day. Children of that age rarely nurse for food, they nurse for comfort, often drifting off to sleep effortlessly after only a few minutes of suckling.

We are in such a rush to have our children grow up, to be first at everything--first to potty train, first to read, etc. We need to slow down and let them enjoy the pleasures of baby-hood, which are all too brief to begin with. You only need ask a child who is old enough to articulate what nursing means to them. My youngest, who nursed until she was almost four, said "Mommy, your milk tastes sweet and makes my tummy feel all warm and snugly." A better endorsement for extended breast-feeding one could not find elsewhere!

I firmly believe that if you implement even a few of these lifestyle changes, not only will your children benefit, but your entire family may also become more peaceful. Manners, civility, politeness and even placing others first are not arcane throwbacks to Victorian times. They are viable tools for allowing us to exist together in tranquility and harmony. Children need to know that their parents care about them. Believe it or not, many teens polled found it most irritating when their parents *didn't* set limits on their activities. Many interpreted this lack of parental authority as a signal that the parents did not really care about what happened to them. Now that is truly frustrating to a young person. My father always had said this about child rearing. "I already love you, there's no disputing that, but I want to raise you so that *others* will love you too."

Towards that end, I believe he was most successful. How many scholars, authors and brilliant minds do you know of who were outstanding contributors to their field, but were complete failures in their personal and family lives? Believe me, it is more the norm among this group than many may realize. I can say as a result of my parents caring so very well for me and taking the time to correct me when it was due that my life has been and is currently exquisitely happy. I have many friends, acquaintances and business partnerships that enrich my life greatly as a result. Most of all I haven't forfeited the joys of marriage and childbearing in lieu of a career as I enjoy the best of both worlds. However, if the choice had to be made between my career and my family, I would choose my family because they indeed have given me the most purpose and joy in life, even beyond measure.

When my children were small, my husband and I

sacrificed for the privilege of me being able to stay home with them. I can remember having very little disposable income then, but my days were so very peaceful, doing projects with the children, taking walks and playing games. The days flew by, but I managed to keep my hand in writing by submitting articles for *The Native Voice*, the newsletter of the New Jersey American Indian Center.

I can say that I have never left a nursing infant, and even took them to class if necessary. What was the result? My students admired my character and conviction to care for my children *myself* and not leave them with sitters. My courses were presented even better than ever because my mind wasn't wandering off, worrying if my baby was all right with a sitter.

Granted, not everyone has a job where they have the option of bringing the child to work with them. Still, we should not close the door on exploring those possibilities if indeed they may be available. What we do for our children, good, bad or indifferent will etch in them impressions for life. Their success and even failure can depend on the way we treat them as children.

These factors reflect a philosophy, not strict medical science, for who can truly validate such matters of the heart? We can, however, look at the examples and mistakes of our generation as well as of our parents. Perhaps in our generation, the pendulum has swung too far to the left, leaving children to decide and supervise their own behavior. This is a big mistake and we are reaping its results.

Ritalin® is not every child's answer. Prozac® is not every teen's solution. We are so inclined to take a pill for everything. Perhaps there is something that can be done to prevent problems in the long run and help a child through difficult times of adjustment. This something, however, has got to start at home. I acknowledge that chemical imbalances in the brain do exist and that for many children and their families, medications such as I have described have been a blessing. Still, the evidence has yet to bear out, at what cost in the long run? Also, how many of these children are more influenced by the stress of social and environmental factors than metabolic dysfunctions? We will forever question ourselves in angst as to whether there was something that could have been done instead of placing the child on medication. We may very well beat ourselves up with guilt if we do not take the time to explore the most comprehensive and safe options for our children's health and well being. This chapter is indeed a good place to start.

Nature's Weeds, Native Medicine has an herbal formula section with products that are safe and natural for young children. A formulation that is of great help to children with hyperactivity and sleepless problems is described as follows:

Children's Natural Calm Blend

> 1/3 cup dried alfalfa leaves
> 1/3 cup dried chamomile
> 1/3 cup dried skullcap

Rich in minerals such as calcium and magnesium that are calming to the nerves, this blend also offers an appreciable amount of B-vitamins that are important to proper central nervous system function. Start off with 1 teaspoon of this blend steeped in 1 cup of water for 3-5 minutes for a weak infusion. It should be used only at bedtime and not in conjunction with other sedative-like medications or cough medicines containing alcohol.

I generally do not recommend giving mineral supplements to young children under the age of 5 years. This is because too much calcium, for example, can damage their maturing kidneys. Children just cannot absorb and assimilate high levels of minerals. Likewise, it is the same issue with fat-soluble vitamins such as vitamin A, D, and E. High amounts of these vitamins can damage the smaller livers of young children.

Hence the best way to supplement is by food choices. Sunflower and sesame seeds are rich in vitamins and minerals (sesame seeds are especially rich in calcium). Wheat germ is loaded with B-complex vitamins and can be added to everything from cereal to meat loaf without much notice.

Cut up, raw, organic vegetables, especially those you grow yourself, are a delight for most little ones. Helping in the garden or even caring for a potted vegetable plant increases the interest in new foods. What child doesn't want to taste something they helped grow from seed?

There is much you can do to help your child eat healthy. Start by setting a good example yourself. Even with the best-laid plans and gourmet meals, remember that children often balk at new foods as a way of asserting their individuality. It also gets the parent's attention, albeit in a negative way. If you don't believe me, just watch your child's eyes light up when you tell your relatives or neighbors, "Oh, Billy just refuses to eat green beans." After a while the list gets even longer as your conversations begin to revolve around Billy and what he *won't* eat. The dinner table becomes a war zone of wills and ultimately the child ends up the loser in health. Once again due to the pressures of the day and too little quality time to spend with the children, many parents just give in to avoid a confrontation.

If a child doesn't like certain foods due to taste and texture, that is perfectly understandable and acceptable. Also, some children are highly allergic and may be picky because they have suffered the consequences of a bad reaction in the past. Once again, this is completely understandable. However, many children will refuse to eat whole food groups such as fruits, vegetables and meats. This is where you will have a serious problem in maintaining proper nutrition for their growing bodies. Given the amount of anorectic children appearing in the pediatrician's office these days, some as young as 5 years old, parents need to be vigilant. These children too often begin by deleting whole food groups from their diet due to "facts" about fat and calorie content. Anorexiais a complex condition that I haven't time to fully discuss here. Yet, I will say that healthy attitudes about food start first with you.

Giving in to your child's power plays at mealtime may only leave him or her on a steady diet of pizza and French fries, foods that will hardly build strong bones and muscles. Sometimes you might just have to be firm and say "This is what the family is eating tonight. Either you eat what we're eating or you don't eat." Trust me, your child will not die from missing one or two meals and there is an important lesson to be learned. The first lesson is that you know more about what is best for them nutritionally. The second lesson is that you are not a short order cook. You or your husband has taken the time to prepare the family meal and out of respect for that effort, children should eat it. Mothers may routinely prepare breakfasts, lunches and dinners to suit each child, which is extremely taxing and time consuming. Teach your children to respect the importance of your time and the fact that you do have a life outside of the kitchen.

These are very simple lessons but they show the child that the universe does not revolve around them. You are also teaching the important concept that in life you cannot expect to have all of your favorite foods prepared all of the time. Likewise you cannot always purchase your favorite clothes, toys, music, etc., either. It is just unrealistic. Trust me, character building begins at the dinner table and teaches children to appreciate what is provided for them.

Prevent Those Back to School Colds

Even though you may have had a wonderfully healthy summer, once school is open you can expect the cold season to begin. In fact, did you know that American children get an average of 6-10 colds per year? In contrast, adults only get about 4 colds per year.

One reason for this difference is the fact that the older we are, the more experienced our immune system becomes at dealing with old "enemy" viruses. The drop off in the amount of colds we get each year is directly proportional to the antibodies we have developed to the most commonly encountered cold viruses.

Just the same there are many things we can do to help our children be healthier during the back to school cold season:

- *Pack a Hand Sanitizer in Their Lunch Box.* The best thing you can do to prevent colds is to wash your hands frequently. Children in school using handrails, doorknobs and lunch tables are exposed to germs that can make them sick. Encourage them to use a hand sanitizer before they eat.
- *Use Lavender Oil to Soothe and Protect.* A few drops of essential oil of lavender can do wonders to naturally calm a squirmy child, but did you know that this essential oil also boosts the immune system? A few drops of Lavender oil on your child's collar will not only help them avoid colds, but will help keep germs at bay.
- *Echinacea Three Weeks On, One Week Off.* You can cycle the Native American herb, *echinacea angustifolia,* in this way to help strengthen your child's immunity. A good brand is Rhino Echinacea™ by Nutrition Now®, which is a raspberry flavored chewable with added vitamin C.
- *Use Zinc Gluconate to Shorten a Cold.* When using about 20 mg per day of zinc, one study noted complete recovery from colds in about 3.9 days, whereas the placebo group took an average of 10.8 days to rebound.

I have used these methods for my own family as well as client/patients with much success. My book, *Nature's Weeds, Native Medicine* has a full section on safe, natural and effective remedies for children.

While there are many herbs casually being added to nutritional supplements for both men and women, I would personally steer clear of them if I were trying to conceive. This is because the initial three months, or the first trimester, is such a dangerous time. Your newly forming baby, whom you may not even be aware of, is highly susceptible to many chemicals, toxins and drugs. Since the neurological system is just beginning to develop during this time, any such intervention can lead to disastrous results. Since this is such a sensitive time for the fetus, I would simply stick with a basic program as has been described in this chapter. Keep in mind also that there are many herbs, too many to list here, that will actually inhibit fertility. Many Native American women used them for thousands of years as just that, an herbal form of contraception. However, this herbal form of birth control is not without a price. Many of these herbs actually poison the system making it uninhabitable for a growing baby. An example of one of these herbs is *wormseed*. All and all it's just not worth the potential damage that can be done to your body by using these toxic herbs. For the purposes of contraception, you would be much better off and healthier choosing another method. The following section will deal with alternatives to birth control pills.

Natural Contraception

Since this section deals with many issues that come up during the childbearing years, I want to offer some alternative ideas to taking birth control pills and explain why you should consider them. Every woman that has a normally functioning endocrine system produces estrogen. The endogenous form (that which is produced by the body) is fully responsible for the development of dominant female characteristics such as rounded hips, enlarging of the breasts and other attributes that define the feminine gender.

From the day that we began our first menstrual cycle until menopause, its presence plays a key role during our reproductive years. If you look at how our bodies are made, the natural state for a woman during her fertile years is to be either pregnant or breast-feeding. Look at the more natural societies, especially Third-World countries. The women often marry very early and begin having children soon after. Often several children are born with perhaps a space of only 18 months between each one. The mother will often breast-feed both her toddler and her newborn at the same time. All of this activity, that is the multiple pregnancies and prolonged lactation, are factors that help decrease the incidence of breast cancer in these societies. You see, it is the constant exposure of the breast and uterine tissues to our own production of estrogen that is of greatest concern. It is thought that maintaining these high levels of estrogen throughout our childbearing years has its price. The correlation between uninterrupted menstrual cycles and increased incidences of breast and uterine cancer is most easily seen in lifestyle differences. Most commonly, a woman who has never been pregnant has an increased risk of developing these female cancers. On the other hand, a woman who conceives and breast-feeds her child decreases her risk by about 37% for the first child, with an additional 17% for each subsequent child. It is the constant barrage of estrogen that is thought to cause the cancerous mutations in the breast and uterine tissues. Drugs like Tamoxifen (Nolvadex®) are used to prevent female cancers from reoccurring due to their ability to block the estrogen receptor sites. This means that your bodies own estrogen can be your own worst enemy.

So this brings us to the subject of natural contraception. Birth control pills contain both estrogen and progesterone. These are exogenous hormones, or those that are produced outside of the body. These drugs have a relatively short track record as compared to other medications. Keep in mind that "the pill" really came into its own as far as widespread use among women in the 1960's. We all know that a woman's incidence of developing cancer increases with age. What will the sixties generation yield as they get older? Time is already telling us quite a bit. One thing that we are hearing is that if you have taken birth control pills for 20 or more years, you may have up to a 40% increased risk for developing a female cancer. Add to this the fact that the incidence of cancer increases with age we may well be seeing such diagnoses at epidemic levels in the near future.

Women need to protect themselves most certainly. An unwanted pregnancy can be catastrophic to a woman who is not physically, emotionally and financially prepared. Subsequently a large number of women are now waiting until they are in their 30's and even 40's to begin a family, citing the same issues. The truth is, the older we are, the less chance we have of conceiving in the first place. These fertility drops are thought to be around 15 to 20% past the age of 35. While there are variations with all individuals, generally the eggs of a woman in her late 30's to mid 40's are not nearly as "fresh" as the eggs that she produced in her twenties. These older eggs also have a greater chance of having chromosomal abnormalities. Hence, despite what the media may portray as miracles of science and modern technology, your best childbearing years may still be ages 25-35.

Chapter 3

THE FULL MOON

The Menopausal Years

Once again, women needn't expect a decline of health and vitality at menopause. For many women it is a liberating time filled with expectations of what *you* want to do as opposed to being a caregiver for everyone else's needs. Nonetheless, you will need to be a little more vigilant about your nutritional status to make sure you get everything you need for this special time in life. Keep in mind that by age 50 or so, many women develop a hiatal hernia. While the cause is not really known, it is suspected that lower production of hydrochloric acid in the stomach causes it to churn more violently in order to disperse the HCL. As a result some of the acid regurgitates or refluxes up into the esophagus. The esophagus, unlike the stomach, has no protective epithelial cells to coat it. Hydrochloric acid in the esophagus is very painful and will eventually erode the sensitive tissue in that area, leading to ulcers. Consuming Tums® is not recommended as it repeats the cycle of neutralizing the HCL, which is needed for proper breakdown of your food's components and digestion.

Menopausal Woman's Nutritional Protocol

Menopausal Woman's Blend

½ cup dried red raspberry leaves and berries

2 tsp. powdered wild yam root

¼ cup dried red clover *leaves* or *Vitex (Chasteberry)*

¼ cup dried chamomile

In this blend the increased amount of wild yam root and the use of red clover *leaves* instead of blossoms help to promote the balance of both estrogen and progesterone. The chamomile is soothing and helps you to relax and get a good night's sleep.

Note: Exclude the red clover leaf component in this formula if you have been diagnosed with an estrogen dependent cancer or are on the prescription drug Tamoxifen.

Additional Nutritional Supplementation

400 mg selenium

Essential fatty acids (1 tbs. flaxseed oil per day)

1,500 mg of calcium

400 mcg folic acid

Osteoporosis Risk Increases after Menopause: Are You Boning Up on Calcium?

Today there are a variety of vitamin supplements on the market. Women require between 1,000 to 1,500 mg of elemental calcium daily to ensure not only optimal bone density but proper heart and neurological function as well. Additionally, after menopause, bone loss accelerates. This can lead to osteoporosis, a serious health problem affecting over 20 million individuals in the United

States and accounts for more than 1 million bone fractures every year.

However, the fact remains that our bodies can only absorb up to 600 mg of calcium at a time; therefore, mega-dosing may do more harm than good. Also, timing is essential. Consuming calcium before bedtime could help ensure that it gets into the bones and is not used up by competing muscle cells trying to displace lactic acid.

Dietary sources are a good place to start, but do not put too much stock in dairy products. Scandinavians are the world's largest consumers of milk products, yet have the highest incidence of osteoporosis. Broccoli, collard greens, sesame seeds and sardines with bones are all appreciably high in absorbable calcium and should be included in our daily menus.

Traditionally Native American women have used *Rubus idaeus,* or red raspberry leaves, as a bio-available source of both calcium and its helper magnesium, along with other trace minerals that are naturally balanced. They also ate fish liver, which is rich in pre-formed vitamin A and D. All of these provided a synergistic approach to building and maintaining bone density well into old age. In fact, I made a point to include my ancestral women's remedies in my book, *Nature's Weeds, Native Medicine,* because of their long track record for efficacy and safety. One cup per day of red raspberry leaf tea will not only give you extra calcium, it will also help facilitate the normal production of estrogen, a factor in accelerated bone loss.

Today especially, it may be difficult to get the right amount of calcium from your diet alone. Other conditions such as low hydrochloric acid in the stomach and aversion or allergies to many calcium-rich foods may make matters worse. Calcium supplements of choice today include calcium citrates and a new substance called microcrystalline apatite, the only form of calcium being reviewed by the FDA for the actual reversal of osteoporosis. (For more information on microcrystalline apatite visit www.miczak.com)

The best advice perhaps might be to take a cue from my Native American ancestors. The combination of diet, exercise, sun and herbs provided a multidirectional approach for a people who had no knowledge or tolerance for milk products or calcium supplements.

Taking Certain Medications Can Cause Nutritional Deficiencies

Long-term medication use is a fact of life for many Americans, especially those over age 65. Menopausal women over age 53 may well be taking several other medications prior to adding estrogen replacement therapy to their existing protocol. Along with the side effects and interactions with other drugs and food supplements, one has to be aware of the risks of developing nutritional deficiencies as a result of using them for extended periods of time.

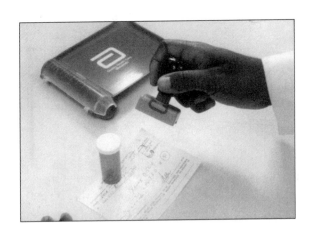

My book, *How Not to Kill Yourself with Deadly Interactions* (Random House), addresses all of these problems head-on with practical solutions to ensure that your health does not suffer as a result of your medication protocol. Here are a few examples taken from the book:

Hormone Replacement Therapy (Estrogens), and Birth Control Pills

These medications stress the body's stores of B-Complex vitamins including folic acid. They are water-soluble vitamins and need to be replaced daily. If you are on any of these therapies or contraceptives and you notice a lack of energy, graying/thinning hair or poor memory, these deficiencies could be at the root of the problem.

Antihistamines

Over-the-counter allergy medications such as Benadryl® and even the new non-sedating antihistamines such as Seldane®, Hismanal® and Claritin® have one thing in common. They all deplete the body of vitamin C. If you use such medications for cold and/or allergy symptoms and you notice that your gums bleed easily from tooth brushing or you bruise easily, you most likely need a little extra vitamin C.

Antibiotics

Medications under this category come in classes of broad and narrow spectrum. Broad-spectrum antibiotics include tetracycline, ampicillin and amoxicillin. What this means is that they kill off both good and bad bacteria indiscriminately, which can lead to stomach problems and yeast infections. The solution is to take some dairy-free lactobacillus acidophilus during the treatment and up to a week after to maintain the balance of intestinal flora.

How Not to Kill Yourself with Deadly Interactions has many more examples of what you can do if you have to take medication long-term. This book is now available by calling toll free 888-795-4274 or through your local bookseller.

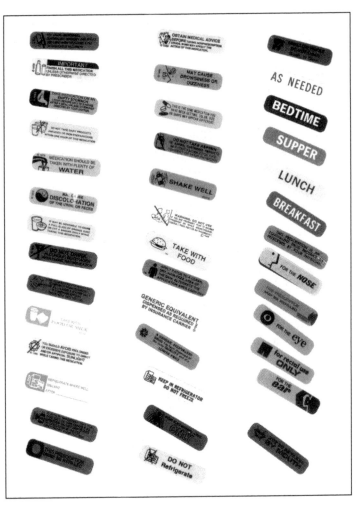

Be sure to heed ags affixed to your medications.

Whereas taking vitamin supplements is often the quickest way to overcome deficiencies, the preferred choice is to get your essential nutrients from food. Why? Because you have a better chance of absorbing natural vitamins and minerals from natural sources than you do from pills.

Remember that your body is simply going into "maintenance mode" during and especially after menopause.

Your body is still producing estrogen through the other organs in your endocrine system such as the thyroid and adrenal glands. This type of estrogen is weaker than the estrogen secreted by your ovaries, which have basically shut down their production. Nonetheless, the weaker form still gets the job done but your body needs time to adjust to it. This is primarily where you will see menopausal symptoms creep in. It is this shift from estrone to estridiol that causes the mood swings, hot flashes, night sweats, forgetfulness and most all of the other symptoms germane to menopause.

Personally, I am not a strong proponent of keeping women on hormone replacement therapy forever, if at all. There is just something quite unnatural about a 70-year-old woman still having her period. Since our chances of developing breast and uterine cancer increase with age, do you really want to add to that risk by taking hormone replacement therapy? We all should think hard and long on that question. Given time, your body will eventually adjust anyway. How many 70-year-old women with or without estrogen replacement are still having hot flashes? Very few, I assure you.

Female Sexual Dysfunction

You should know that you do not have to be menopausal to experience female sexual dysfunction, which is by definition a woman's inability to experience full arousal and orgasm. While only about 25% of all women experience orgasm during intercourse, many women have never experienced an orgasm at all. There are many contributing factors as to why sexual fulfillment may be more difficult as we approach menopause.

While testosterone is generally thought to be the hormone responsible for libido, or sex drive, other hormones play their part as well. In any event, we begin to produce less of *all* sex hormones as we age. This may not totally be a bad thing. Centuries of bombardment by estrogen on receptor cells, especially those of the breasts, seem to increase the possibility of mutations at the cellular level. This is why a woman's risk of getting breast cancer increases with age. That withstanding, drops in estrogen can lead to vaginal dryness and loss of elasticity in the vaginal wall. This can make intercourse dreadfully uncomfortable and most certainly not something to look forward to! Also, when we are younger, we have a natural boost courtesy of our menstrual cycle. When we ovulate, the vaginal mucus secretions change in viscosity and assist in lubrication. Likewise, blood flow to the genital area in general is optimal. As we get older and perhaps have not watched our cholesterol, lack of blood profusion and circulation can show up even in this very delicate area. Another reason to watch your HDL and LDL ratios of cholesterol, right?

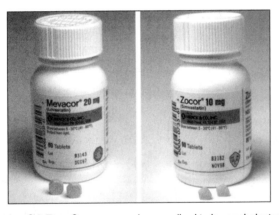

Mevacor® & Zocor® are commonly prescribed to lower cholesterol.

Other studies reveal that once a woman completes menopause, her sense of smell is not as keen as it was during her childbearing years. Don't feel bad. Pre-pubescent girls share this same handicap. Their sense of smell develops to its highest level once they menarche, or have their first menstrual cycle. It is thought that sexual desire is in part triggered by our sense of smell, specifically by our primitive ability to pick up pheromones emitted from the opposite sex. These odiferous glands are located in the armpits (sounds appealing), around the nipples and the genital area of both sexes. When exposed to these pheromones, we receive a chemical signal that the other person is interested in us. That in and of itself assists in sexual arousal.

It is a given we are dealt a few physical limitations during menopause. Have no fear as there are many practical solutions available. First of all, if you are noticing a sudden decrease in sexual desire, pay a visit to your doctor. Have you just started a new medication? Certain medications such as those prescribed for hypertension and depression can have terrible sexual side effects. The problem can leave as quickly as it appeared once you change your medication. In other cases, lack of interest in life in general can cloud one's outlook. Depression, loss, isolation and anxiety all take their toll. Once again, it is important to address the underlying problem first to see if there is an improvement. Fine. Let's say you are healthy, nothing is bothering you and you are not on any problematic medications. So what's wrong? Well, just as men may have erectile problems, so can be the case with women. If blood flow to the clitoris, which corresponds to the male penis, is poor you may find it difficult to sense arousal and experience orgasm. However, other factors such as a mate who does not allow enough foreplay for this to take place is surely a major part of the problem. The issue is when everything is normal, but sexual interest and satisfaction still eludes you, it is time to look at some options. Internet offers for "Spanish Fly" should be avoided like the Plague! Real Spanish Fly was used by livestock farmers looking to increase their herd. Spanish Fly is actually a genital irritant that causes blood flow of inflammatory proportions. The poor bulls are simply trying to rid themselves of the torment! Does this sound like something you would like to experience?

I can suggest something that works and is safe. There are several brands of gels and cremes on the market that contain the amino acid L-arginine. L-arginine is one of the building blocks of protein and is completely harmless. These gels are applied directly to the genital area, specifically the clitoris, to facilitate an erection and sensitivity. Obviously products such as these work on men as well, but our focus here is on the female anatomy. With a clitoral erection in place, the entire area becomes very sensitive and orgasm is much easier to achieve. Some of these products combine menthol with the L-arginine for added absorption and stimulation. The result is said to be a "cool burn," which will usually not irritate sensitive personal areas if used as directed. If vaginal dryness is a contributing factor, there are your stand-by gels such as K-Y® jelly. However, newer versions have added vitamin E and other lubricants that help reduce the effects of estrogen loss in the area. Many women also use progesterone crème derived from wild yam, which helps balance hormonal depletion. Prescription products may utilize hormones, but you may not need that level of therapy. Try something less invasive first, but in my opinion it may be safer to simply use a hormone replacement crème in the *area of need* as opposed to the systemic use of such drugs. You have less chance of other organs such as breast tissue being stimulated as a result.

Gel preparations with L-arginine and menthol such as *Viagel*® and *Viacreme*® are relatively easy to use and most women notice a difference with the first application. L-arginine is an amino acid and is the basic building block of the Nitric Oxide pathway. Simply put, when applied the L-arginine stimulates the tissue surfaces causing dilation of the blood vessels in the clitoris. This is why administration of the gel is made directly to the bare clitoris. You will need to gently retract the clitoral hood and apply the gel to the site. Reapply as often as needed or desired. Many women report ease of multiple orgasms and relief of vaginal dryness while using gels containing L-arginine.

Female Incontinence

As we age, our pelvic muscles begin to lose their tone, especially if we are not engaging in sexual activity as frequently as we have in the past. The sad fact is that there are very few activities other than intercourse that will actually keep these muscles in shape. Diminished lubrication and elasticity of vaginal tissues may make intercourse less of a frequent affair, but my previous recommendations should offer much relief. These same muscles used during copulation also allow us to control ourselves long enough to make it to the bathroom with a full bladder. Many women may not have a problem holding themselves until they can get to a restroom only to be surprised when a sudden stream of urine gushes out after a sneeze!

Everyday activities such as laughing, coughing or even hugging can trigger what is known as "stress incontinence." When put under stress, the muscles cannot hold up enough to control urination. Although common, incontinence of any kind merits further tests and investigation by your doctor. Incontinence can be a sign of a more serious underlying medical condition.

We see so many commercials for Poise® and Depends® that we assume incontinence is a normal part of aging. Not really. While there are many bizarre tools and gadgets that promise to exercise the pelvic muscles that control urinary flow, most are useless. You can get the very same toning for free by doing *Kegel* exercises. This exercise is named for the doctor who first isolated these muscles in the female anatomy. They make up and support the pelvic floor and often lose their tone after childbirth. Kegel exercises are simple and easy to implement into your everyday routine.

Each time you go to the bathroom to urinate, try stopping and starting your urinary stream several times, each time holding it as long as you can. For example, begin your urine stream and then do a Kegel exercise for 3 seconds, release and repeat the sequence. Gradually increase the time your urine flow is stopped to 4 seconds, 5 seconds, and so on. The point is to familiarize yourself with the muscles of the pelvic region and what role they play in bladder control. Another added bonus is that by strengthening the pelvic floor, problems of female sexual dysfunction will also abate because these are the same muscles that are involved in the muscle contractions that make up the female orgasm. If your Kegel muscles lack strength, so will your orgasms when you can have them. The connection is evident. The more toned your pelvic floor is, the easier it will be to climax and the stronger your orgasms will become. With a little exercise you might not need the Depends® after all!

Breast Health For Life

I would like to briefly address the issue of breast cancer, the incidence of which increases with age. The timetable for mammograms has been rolled back. It is now recommended that women have them once yearly after age 40. Previously it was recommended to begin them around age 50. While I am not going to go into the politics behind this change in testing, I will say that during your menstruating years, breast tissue is constantly changing primarily due to the influences of estrogen. You know, that swelling that occurs near your period? The lumpiness of your breasts because you indulged in just a little too much chocolate this month? These changes bring about flags that often result in false positives in mammograms. Many women are put through unnecessary mental and emotional anguish with very little reward in regard to protecting themselves from breast cancer. Not only that, you are adding 10 more years of radiation exposure to your breast tissue without any concrete assurance that the mammogram will detect breast cancer or that you will survive it any better. It is my personal opinion that for *most* women, a yearly mammogram starting at age 50 is still the better route.

If you have a family history of breast cancer in that you have a first degree relative (your mother or sister), who developed breast cancer, especially before the age of 50, then your testing protocol will be quite different. Also women with massive breasts or who are Jewish tend to be at a higher risk. In these instances, testing may be advisable at an even earlier phase than is recommended for the general population. Some women with a genetic link to the disease have even opted to have both breasts removed prophylactically before breast cancer has been detected. While this is entirely up to the woman, you can see how serious this problem really is.

If you suspect that you may be at risk for developing breast cancer, there are things that you can do now. Diet is a major factor next to genetics. However, before you run out and buy soy and tofu everything, there is something you should know. While preliminary studies may suggest soy products are helpful in preventing breast cancer, *if you have already been diagnosed with breast cancer too much soy can pose other problems* such as can be seen in two case studies from my own nutritional consulting practice:

Over-consumption of soy products can lead to iron deficiency anemia.

Case #356

A vegetarian or vegan woman in her 30's who consumed no animal products such as dairy or eggs presented with lethargy, inability to focus or concentrate and irritability. She said that her protein intake consisted mostly of soy products including soy milk and soy cheese. After reading the results of her complete blood count with differential, it was noted that the hematology analyzer

(Becton Dickenson's QBC Autoread Plus) indicated a diagnosis of iron deficiency anemia. Soy products block the absorption of iron. The patient took an organic non-constipating iron supplement apart from her food. This formula also contained vitamin C to help her absorb the iron better. After four months she was tested again. Her hemoglobin and hematocrit readings registered within normal limits.

Over-consumption of soy products can interfere with thyroid function.

Case #502

One case study showed a woman diagnosed with hypothyroidism who was experiencing trouble managing her condition after introducing soy products into her diet. She was consuming 3-4 servings of soy per day as supplied in soy milk, tofu cheese and regular fat tofu.

Over time she began noticing weight gain, lethargy, thinning hair and dry skin, which are all symptoms consistent with a hypoactive thyroid even though she was on medication (Synthroid®, levothyroxine). Her doctor was about to increase her dose when I suggested that she cut out the soy products to see if this would help. After about a month of discontinuance, her symptoms began to abate and her thyroid panel tests were found to be within normal ranges again. It appears that the phytoestrogen activity of soy competes with the same receptors shared by the thyroid medication. This may cause a person to require higher amounts of thyroid medication to function normally.

Far more sinister is the misunderstanding regarding the health benefits associated with soy, specifically for women who have had breast cancer already. Many women turn to soy during the menopausal years hoping to both quell symptoms associated with the change of life and prevent breast cancer. Before you venture forth on a soy and tofu rich diet, consider the following:

The Skinny on Soy

The Benefits, the Risks

Soybean production in the U.S. is at an all time high. Soy is used in animal feed, cosmetics, dyes, food and beverages... the list just goes on and on. Women who are perimenopausal (near menopause) swear by it for relief of menopausal symptoms. This is because of soy's documented phytoestrogen effects. Phytoestrogens are literally translated as "plant estrogens."

Phytoestrogens are not to be dismissed as ineffective because they are derived from a vegetable source. Not at all! Phytoestrogens are much weaker than the endogenous estrogens, or those made by our own bodies. All the same they are powerful enough to trigger the natural turnover of our own body's estrogen. This is preferable in many ways to estrogen replacement therapy, especially if you are at high risk of developing female cancers. People in this category would usually be women with at least one first-degree relative who has had breast or uterine cancer. Use of phytoestrogens in lieu of estrogen replacement therapy might be a preferred method if these are your circumstances.

This brings us to the subject of soy. Soybeans (*Glycinemax*) are a member of the *pulse* family. *They are toxic if not prepared and processed properly*. The many cultures of Asia, where soybeans have been used as a primary source of protein, figured this out over 5,000 years ago. Right now, there are over 2,500 varieties of soybeans in cultivation, some containing more protein than others. They yield more than just a food crop. Soybeans are used in everything from inks to the making of plastics! Highly versatile, soybeans give us soybean oil, soy sauce, soy milk, tofu and are even used as a coffee substitute. However, I wouldn't toss out the Folgers® just yet. It is one of the best sources of phytoestrogens around. In fact, eating just two servings of tofu a day (8 oz of soy milk and

4 oz of tofu), has been shown to relieve hot flashes, lower cholesterol and even increase bone density. Soy is also the only vegetable that contains Omega-3 essential fatty acids. These essential fats allow for the ease of synthesization, or production of, estrogen. An added benefit of soy is that it is believed to help decrease the risk of breast cancer *but only if you do not already have it.* Keep this in mind and we will return to this point later.

The problem with getting the benefit of soy is in compliance. You will need at least 2-3 servings of soy per day to get the results as described previously. If you do not come from a culture that traditionally cooks with tofu, this might be hard to swallow (pardon the pun). You might get around this problem by simply using a concentrated soy powder that can be blended into cereal, juice, milk or a shake as will soon be described. You will also need to take note of the fat content. Whole soy milk is very fattening, as many of my female clients/patients have already discovered. It isn't unusual to see a gain of 4–5% body fat after only two or three months on whole soy milk. If you want to "have your soy and eat it too," make sure you choose the lower fat versions in both the milk and tofu.

Now the down side to soy. *If you have already been diagnosed with cancer, especially a female cancer, do not take, eat or use soy products.* It appears that something in the soy triggers the activation of preexisting cells. I have actually witnessed this several times in my own private practice. A woman with breast cancer will go through chemotherapy, medication, tamoxifen, everything. She will finally go into remission and then say, "I hear tofu can help prevent breast cancer so I will start eating lots of it!" Wrong, wrong, wrong. As I have said before, use of soy products may be of benefit *before* you develop an active cancer. However once you have it the use of soy may only work to reestablish it. One woman who came to visit me for a healthy eating program did just this. She was doing fine, but eating tons of tofu while in remission.

Upon her next visit, the doctors noted her breast cancer had returned. The only thing that she had done differently with her diet was to add tofu. A sad lesson to be learned. After all that she had been through, she was back at square one. If this information helps but one woman, I have done my job.

Hair Loss Due to Hormone Depletion or Chemotherapy

This is a sensitive issue, especially for women. You see, we are not expected to lose our hair. This is why some types of hair loss are referred to as "male pattern" baldness. However, many women actually experience the same thing. Hereditary factors, sudden drops in estrogen, chemotherapy and emotional crisis can rob us of our crowning glory.

Before you run out and expose yourself to costly solutions that may do more harm than good, please read the following interview with Kimberly Belk, RN. Nurse Belk speaks with personal experience regarding how she was able to deal with her own hair loss problem as well as help other women in similar circumstances. She is a forward-thinking businesswoman with ample sincere empathy for her clients, which helps put them at ease with this devastating problem.

Q. What is your medical education/professional background?

A. I began my career as a volunteer nursing assistant in 1968, worked my way up the ranks from there to an EMT, LPN and then a RN. I started college in San Diego, studied my way back east, and graduated with my nursing degree from Augusta College, now called Augusta State University, which is part of the University of Georgia system. I also hold two advanced certifications in nursing as a Certified Rehabilitation Registered Nurse and a Certified Case Management Nurse.

Q. What personal life experiences led you to start Belk and Associates, Inc.?

A. I personally suffer hair loss in the form of androgenetic alopecia, which I first noticed at age 32. Several years ago, I made a very foolish decision to try bonding a hairpiece to my head, which resulted in an allergic reaction to the glue. This decision only made the alopecia worse and now I wear a wig or hairpiece daily. The cost of a quality wig or hairpiece astounded me so much that I decided that something had to be done to make these products affordable. Also, the salespeople and stylists I spoke with did not seem to be well informed on the many types of hair replacement products available.

Q. What is your business philosophy?

A. If I won't put a product on my own head, I am certainly not going to put it on someone else's head. My customers look to me to guide them and I will not betray that trust. This business is not about making a living; it is about making a difference in the lives of those who suffer hair loss. The majority of people who wear wigs and hairpieces are not wearing them as a fashion statement; it is based on need, and to take advantage of someone in this situation of desperation is a sin, in my opinion. I see my involvement in the hair replacement industry as an extension of my career as a nurse; I serve God by serving His children.

Q. As a nurse, what correlation have you seen between a female patient's personal appearance effecting their overall mental outlook and recovery?

A. When a woman thinks she looks bad, she feels worse. It's that simple. Women who are able to put on their make-up, comb their hair or wig, and wear a nice, comfortable outfit have a more positive outlook. Even if she is only going into the kitchen to have dinner with her family, the sense of well being gained from "looking good" is priceless. This phenomenon is supported by scientific fact, and this also is the basis of the "Look Good, Feel Better" program through the American Cancer Society. Both men and women become adversely affected by a negative self-image. And, it has been documented in medical literature that prayer improves the likelihood of recovery, whether prayers are said by or for the patient.

Q. What special services do you offer to your wig customers? For example, consultation on suitable types of wig hair, fitting tips, etc.

A. I like to get to know my customers and have a feel for their lifestyle, their habits and their personal sense of fashion. I discuss with my customers the various types of wigs, types of hair, types of attachments and sizes available, different kinds of hairstyles, and how long they expect to wear the wig. This information is then used to guide the customer to an appropriate choice for them. I also offer salon services for styling and cutting their wig if their personal stylist is not comfortable performing these services for them.

Q. What do you see in the future for Belk and Associates, Inc.?

A. God willing, I plan to continue to provide these services until I am physically unable to serve those in need. I also plan to keep abreast of new developments in the industry so that I can inform my customers of the best options available to meet their needs.

Q. Do you ship overseas?

A. At this time, I have never shipped overseas, but I have

made inquiries on the processes involved with such transactions and will implement whatever policies needed to accomplish those transactions.

Q. Are you considering a page translator for international language sales?

A. Yes, if my host will support it.

Q. What is your website address?

A. www.belkwigs.com and www.accenthair.com

Q. Why should a woman purchase a wig on-line from Belk and Associates, Inc.?

A. As someone who has suffered hair loss, I am empathetic to those who are also suffering. I went through a difficult time emotionally dealing with my hair loss, and an even worse time trying to find a suitable hair replacement that looked natural. I understand the heartbreak associated with hair loss and would gladly spare anyone those feelings. I also want my customers, above all else, to be satisfied with their looks. Nothing can replace what God gave us, but with proper understanding, a reasonable replacement can be found. Sometimes, it takes time and patience, but I never give up hope that I can help someone.

I have personally seen women with extreme hair loss going about their day to day business. I know it must make them feel self-conscious because I feel uncomfortable for them! We're just not used to the sight of a balding woman. In fact, the Nazi German concentration camps intentionally shaved the heads of the female prisoners to make them feel more vulnerable. In many ancient societies, a woman will cut her hair to denote mourning or remorse.

Long, thick, healthy hair is often associated with inner health and beauty. A woman may feel perfectly fine, but genetics or her hormones may have dealt her an unfair blow. It is sad that her outer persona does not reflect the youth and vibrancy within. This goes way beyond vanity. When we look our best, we are able to concentrate on more important things. I will give you an example that we all can relate to. You have to give a speech in front of a large group of people. Suddenly you get a dollop of mustard right on the front of your white blouse! No time to clean it, you have to give your discourse NOW. What are you going to be thinking about? Your delivery and connecting with your audience? Most likely not. You are going to be worried that everyone is looking at that mustard smear instead of listening to you. While most of the time we are far more concerned about such things than our audience, it is an issue to consider.

I have had many enriching experiences in life. For example, did you know that I was a model and in a major beauty pageant? Yes indeed! I still model for my articles and book covers, but obviously what is going on here is more substance related. Still, packaging doesn't hurt. Even if you are not the victim of hair loss, you can use hair additions and wigs to change or enhance your looks. Wigs made of 100% European hair will be soft, natural and nearly undetectable as a wig. The *GeorGie* line is the best example of this type of high-end wig as they are gorgeous, yet affordable. Belk Associates carries GeorGie wigs, which far and away are the absolute best that money can buy. You will be amazed at how beautiful and natural they are as they are virtually undetectable as hair-pieces.

It is quite normal to care about your appearance. In many nursing homes and hospitals, elderly patients are often charted for progress with the "Lipstick Test." This is quite simple. Upon feeling better a female patient will ask for a hand mirror, a brush and some lipstick. Caring about one's personal appearance is a sign of physical and emotional health. Health providers often encourage patients who have sustained serious injuries to get up, get dressed and apply a bit of makeup, which makes the patient look and feel better.

Many hospitals now have annexed organizations that will fit female cancer patients with prosthetic breasts, wigs, etc. Actually, whatever they need to make them feel whole again, just as they were before their illness. This is very important. Preliminary studies indicate that women who receive this kind of support have a better patient outcome than those who give up and take no interest in their appearance or life in general. The saying is that if you look good you will feel good. While not entirely sci-entific, there are areas of the human psyche that we still do not understand.

Chapter 4

WEIGHT CONTROL

Why Your Scale May Be Lying

I t is a known fact that we Americans squander billions of dollars each year on worthless diet pills, foods and programs that just do not work. In fact, recent government surveys show that up to 55% of us are overweight. As a health concern, even being slightly obese significantly increases an individual's risk of coronary heart disease, diabetes and even some types of cancer. Many health experts classify obesity as being 20% over your ideal body weight using the Body Mass Index, which indicates in theory what you should weigh for your height and gender. Many diet centers still use this method because it is inexpensive and simple.

The Body Mass Index chart, however, does not calculate what percentage of you is lean muscle mass and how much is fat. Adding to the confusion, many are more interested in quantitative losses, not qualitative. In other words if you have recently lost 15 lb through dieting, you have probably lost 15 lb of muscle, or the active tissue that burns calories. Also bear in mind that muscle weighs almost twice as much as fat, although it is more compact. For example, a weight lifter may have the perfect physique but is considered "overweight" according to the

Body Mass Index method. This is why the numbers on your bathroom scale may be misleading you.

Measuring your percentage of body-fat is a much more accurate way to determine overall health and physical fitness. Women ages 18-29 do well between 17-24% body-fat whereas females over the age of 30 should be between 20-27%.

Young men under age 30 can range 14-20% body-fat while those over 30 need to stay within the 17-23% limits. The difference allowed each gender in regard to healthy body-fat lies within the need for hormonal production and regulation. A female's extra body-fat facilitates the manufacture of estrogen. This is why female athletes with very low body-fat percentages may cease having their menstrual cycles altogether. In fact, some fat is needed by both genders to make the neurotransmitter serotonin, which protects the kidneys and maintains normal hormone levels.

Here are a few tips to make sure your losses are really gains in health:

1) Always include exercise as part of your weight loss program. If you don't, the weight you lose will be muscle.

2) Be sure to get enough high quality protein. Turkey, chicken breast, tuna packed in water, egg whites and legumes contain the amino acids needed to build and maintain healthy muscle tissue.

3) Snack! Graze on 5-6 "mini-meals" per day. This will raise your calorie-burning rate much higher than if you eat only 3 large meals a day.

There are many diet pills available over the counter that may not be very safe or effective. Steer clear of Ma

Huang, also known as Chinese ephedra, or guarana. These herbs have amphetamine-like components that can make you jittery, induce high blood pressure and insomnia.

Another product often added to "natural" weight loss pills is the very unnatural phenylpropanolamine hydro-chloride found in common supermarket and drug store products such as Dexatrim®. If you read the back of the box it cautions you not to take this product if you have or are being treated for:

Depression	Heart disease
An eating disorder	Diabetes
Enlarged prostate	Thyroid disease
High blood pressure	Insomnia

Additionally, you should not use weight control products with the active ingredient phenylpropanolamine if you are taking the following over-the-counter or prescription medications:

- Cough/cold or allergy medications containing any form of phenylpropanolamine

- Any oral nasal decongestant

- A prescription monoamine oxidase inhibitor (MAOI) for depression

The Medical Letter, a highly respected drug therapy publication, states "Phenylpropanolamine and related drugs have prominent effects on the sympathetic nervous system and should not be used by individuals suffering from diabetes, hypertension, heart disease or thyroid disease without seeking medical advice."

Adding to this the American Medical Association has stated that phenylpropanolamine containing diet products are only "minimally effective." Since this compound is available over the counter in many commercial and "holistic" diet products, they tend to be abused most by teenagers, especially young girls. You do not need a prescription or parental consent to purchase them right off the shelf, increasing the potential for misuse.

Instead, you might wish to use these natural weight loss food supplements to help you lose fat and increase your calorie-burning rate:

- Fucus or Seaweed (Bladderwrack):

  Kelp, nori and other sea "veggies" are rich in organic iodine, which is necessary for normal thyroid function. Kelp is also a gentle diuretic useful in the safe and effective relief of excess water weight gain. (**Note:** *Do not use if you have diabetes.*)

- Chitin or Chitosan:

  Harvested from shrimp and lobster shells, chitin readily binds with dietary fats in the intestine, preventing their absorption. Taken 20-30 minutes before a meal it also helps you to eat less by making you feel full. As an added bonus, chitin may also have a beneficial effect towards lowering cholesterol. (**Note:** *Do not take if you are allergic to shellfish.*)

- Pyruvate:

  This compound is related to pyruvic acid, which is found naturally in the body. Pyruvate is a direct salt of ester of pyruvic acid. Studies suggest that pyruvate plays an important role in the body's process that converts carbohydrates and fats into fuel or energy. Pyruvic acid is produced in the body and serves as an intermediate product in the metabolism of carbohydrates, fats and amino acids. Most studies recommend 2,000 to 3,000 mg, or 2-3 grams, of pyruvate per day for best results.

- Chromium Picolinate:

  Most Americans are deficient in this trace mineral because the soils no longer contain it. Crops do not need chromium to grow, so we do not notice that this key element is even missing. Chromium is important because it is essential in the metabolism of glucose, or "sugar." It also helps the body burn fat thereby increasing the muscle to fat ratio. By adding leaner muscle tissue, you can naturally eat more, yet burn more calories since muscle is active tissue, and always "hungry" for fuel to burn. A daily allowance of 200 mcg of chromium picolinate (chromium chelated with picolinate, a naturally formed amino acid metabolite) per day is considered safe. Another form of this trace mineral is chromium nicotinate, which is simply chromium bound to nicotinic acid. This form is also very effective but one should note that there might be a slight flushing from the niacin component when using this form.

- L-Arginine:

  Amino acids are the building blocks of every protein in every cell of the body. L-arginine is just one of them but it plays a major role in helping your anterior pituitary release growth hormone while you sleep. Products that provide L-arginine along with other amino acids, aloe vera and chitosan in a liquid form are very absorbable.

By tying all of this together, you can begin to build your own supplemental protocol according to your own specific needs and goals. Each New Year one of the top resolutions on everyone's list is to lose weight and shape up. Nonetheless, Americans are still some of the most overweight people in the world.

Native American people worked hard to chase down and grow food, which was sometimes sparse. For example, the month of February was often known as the "hunger moon." This was the time when many of the foods stored for winter had run out. It was also too early to get much game from hunting or food from the garden. Many tribes experienced hunger and even starvation, depending on the severity of the conditions.

There is a theory that certain people may be genetically able to withstand long periods of hunger better than others. This is the "starvation gene" theory. People with such genetic traits may be able to survive on less food than other people of similar weight and activity. It appears that the body stores more by way of fat from the same sampling of calories. Fat can then be burned as fuel for the body's energy requirements during lean times when meals may be few and far between.

Today in America, many have easy access to high calorie, rich dishes including fast foods. Those who may have inherited the "starvation gene" as a way of survival may find themselves putting on excess pounds of fat by consuming these foods. We can see this among many tribes of the Southwest. The Piutes, for example, have high incidences of obesity and diabetes. We are witnessing this happening with other tribes as well. It is often seen among those who have left their traditional native foods for processed fast foods never eaten by their ancestors.

So what can you do apart from avoiding the fast food fat trap? Well, you will need to boost your body's metabolic rate, or the speed by which your body burns calories. This will prevent food calories from being stored as adipose tissue or fat. Another secret to long term weight control is to increase your muscle to fat ratio. Lean muscle is active and burns more calories than fat, which just sits there and does nothing!

Although we begin to lose lean muscle tissue at a rate of about 1-2% per year past age 30, a weight training regime can begin to offset that loss. Remarkably, one well published study including men over the age of 60 and young men in their 20's found no distinct difference in either group's ability to add lean muscle mass. The older male participants showed steady gain in response to their weight lifting program, concluding that muscle fitness can be improved at *any* age. This also applies to women.

Weight lifting is a low impact exercise. While it does not build the same level of cardiovascular health as aerobics, it can and should be a part of any cross training program. Low weights and multiple repetitions will tone while high weights with fewer "reps" will build size and add bulk. Another perk is that weight bearing exercise places positive stress on the skeletal system, increasing bone mass, strength and density. In fact, one of the main factors that predisposes a person to osteoporosis is a sedentary lifestyle, which no amount of calcium pills can repair.

To support your body's ability to burn rather than store calories as fat we can look to our helpful herbs. While you should avoid stimulating herbs containing caffeine, ephedrine (Ma Huang) or guarana, there are some herbs that will work with your body to help you slim down naturally. Here is one such formula taken from my book *Nature's Weeds, Native Medicine:*

Slimming Tea Blend

½ cup dried watercress

½ cup dried kelp

¼ cup dried chamomile flowers

The watercress and kelp contain naturally occurring, organic iodine which is crucial to the proper function of the thyroid. A sluggish or mildly hypoactive thyroid can show up as unexplained weight gain, dry skin and thinning hair as well as an extreme sensitivity to coldness. As an added bonus, this formula has a mild diuretic action, which helps control excess water weight gain we women may experience as part of PMS.

Note: If you have diabetes, do not use the kelp component in this formula since kelp has been known to increase blood sugar in diabetics.

One thing to remember is to eat at least 4-5 mini-meals per day. Why? Well, your body will burn these smaller meals much more quickly than 3 larger ones. So, snacking is good! Smaller, frequent meals will boost your metabolic rate and allow you to eat normally without starving yourself. Once again, lean muscle tissue is active and always "hungry." This is due to the fact that muscle is always contracting and burning calories as a result.

As you "cut up," dropping excess body fat, you will find that your clothes will fit better. Even though the numbers on your bathroom scale may not change dramatically, you will soon notice a slimmer, more toned silhouette in the mirror.

Chapter 5

S L E E P   T O   R E N E W

Every night, our bodies and minds are given the extraordinary opportunity to rebuild and renew. A restful night's sleep can be regarded as one of the most valuable gifts one can hope to attain. Many factors weigh into why we tend to have more sleep disturbances as we grow older. There is the diminishing of specific hormones that facilitate achieving complete sleep, which would include the R.E.M. phase, or rapid eye movement, portion of the cycle. R.E.M. sleep is associated with the dream cycle. Without it, we cannot have a truly refreshing and rejuvenating night's rest. We need to dream! There are other factors such as nutritional deficiencies that can deprive one of R.E.M. sleep. For example, if you are not getting enough B complex vitamins, R.E.M. cycle sleeping is sure to evade you. Other factors include getting enough calcium and magnesium BEFORE going to bed. If taken too early, these minerals are simply utilized by active muscle. It is far better to take your calcium supplement after dinner and just prior to bed in the amount of no more than 500 mg at a time. This is because our body really cannot absorb more than 500 mg of elemental calcium in one dose. Your nervous system requires both calcium and magnesium to function properly as well.

Likewise, the drop in production of melatonin, estrogen and growth hormone all play a major role in the increased incidences of sleep disorders in middle-aged to older adults.

The expression "sleeping like a baby" is well-founded in scientific study and research. This is because the anterior pituitary secretes growth hormone during the deepest phase of our sleep cycle. This would be during the time when our brain waves adopt the Alpha configuration, which is associated with the deepest level of relaxation. So the old wives' tale that says, "when the baby is sleeping, it is growing" is actually quite accurate.

As we age, our pituitary glands do not secrete as much growth hormone as before. It is still there; however, getting it to work for us is now more of a challenge. I would advise against taking growth hormone shots or supplements. This is because of something called homeostasis. When the body detects a certain level of hormone present in the bloodstream, it begins to shut down the natural production of the same hormone from your endocrine glands. For example, if you have been taking Synthroid® for more than two or three years for an under-active thyroid, most likely your body and thyroid have specifically adjusted to having the hormone provided for it. The thyroid that does not need to produce very much thyroxine will slowly begin to shut down, shrink and atrophy. It has received the signal that its services for the production of thyroid hormones is no longer needed. The body is very stingy about producing hormones without demand, therefore that which is not needed, wanes.

Rather than take questionable hormones to replace those that are starting to lag in production consider this. There are natural supplements that can *facilitate* the release of growth hormone, which is already present in the pituitary. In addition, there are activities that can force the release of growth hormone naturally.

First let's discuss the supplements. You need only first look towards the building blocks of protein called amino acids. Essential amino acids are those that the body cannot make on its own but must be supplied in the daily diet. The trick is to get protein into the cells, which is somewhat the function that growth hormone has on our bodies when we are younger. This is why young people can eat a seemingly endless variety of fats, starches and sugars and still maintain a lean muscle mass overall. One of the things that you can do to assist the release of growth hormone while you sleep is to take liquid or gel-capped amino acids just before bed. A full complement of the amino acids is recommended; however, it is the L-arginine that has the most potential for this application. Whichever amino acid supplement you choose, make sure that L-arginine is present. I like to recommend the liquid form of these amino acids over hard-pressed pills and tablets because they are instantly absorbed. When taken just before bed on an empty stomach (two to three hours after your last meal or snack), they are easily assimilated, since amino acids are well absorbed in the presence of food.

You will find yourself achieving a much more complete and restful sleep cycle with the added benefit of your own natural growth hormone to complement the night. Within a month you will notice leaner, more defined muscles, thicker skin and a diminishing of fine lines and wrinkles. After three months, you should notice a marked difference and improvement in your muscle tone, fat loss and overall rejuvenated appearance.

The second way to encourage the release of your body's own growth hormone is the old-fashioned way. That would be hard, long and sustained aerobic and anaerobic exercise. Body builders like Arnold Schwarzenegger used to train very hard using low repetitions with very high weights in their exercise routine. This kind of stress on the muscle builds mass and bulk. Yet this intensive training brought about something else. That was the release of growth hormone, which announced its presence in a very unique way. Most hard-core body builders would have a bucket near their workout equipment. During the most intense phase of the weight lifting session, the body builders would be seen vomiting into these pails! The nausea that they felt was due to the rapid release of growth hormone during hard exercise and lifting. I myself have noticed a similar sensation after many hours of intense in-line skating. If you are not into weights you can choose another way to get your daily dose of growth hormone, but be advised that you have to turn up the intensity either way to get results. No, a casual stroll around the block won't quite do it. You need to be pushing the limits for quite some time to get similar results, but they are well worth it.

I have devoted a complete chapter in this book to exercises such as biking and in-line skating, both of which are my absolute favorites for cardiovascular toning, burning fat and toning the muscles. Regular, vigorous exercise will also surely set you up for a good night's sleep, guaranteed. If you haven't exercised in a long time, check with your doctor first to get the go-ahead.

It goes without saying that you need the best possible "equipment" in order to reach your goal of a good night's rest for renewal and rejuvenation. There are two items that many of my patients have used with much success and I have personally tested to my own satisfaction. The first item that every bed must have is light, warm covers that do not restrict circulation, but allow the body to maintain its own comfortable temperature. Apart from using breathable materials such as cotton and silk for your bedding, you should invest in a good quality goose down comforter. As a child I had the pleasure of sleeping under one on overnight visits at my Aunt Sylvia's house. It was an utter bliss and I was never cold. Comforters made of both goose down and the more expensive eiderdown have been used since before medieval times, especially in England. There are primitive records and drawings showing the down of ducks and geese being sprinkled between the bed sheets in English cottages. Later on, they were sewn into fabric and the duvet was born. Today a wide variety of goosedown comforters are available to fit most every budget. The only extra expense you will incur after purchasing the comforter is the need for a duvet cover. This is simply to keep the comforter clean and looks much like a large pillowcase with buttons to keep it closed and secured over your duvet and that is it. I have slept with nothing else on my bed; that is no extra blankets, quilts, etc. for the past eight years, winter through summer. The air-trapping quality of the goose down naturally regulates your own body's heat and temperature despite the coldest nights and conditions.

For those with diabetes or fibromyalgia, light but warm bedding that does not restrict circulation to the lower extremities is a godsend. You simply loft or fluff the comforter before getting into bed to increase the warmth capacity. When shopping for a new goose down comforter, be sure that the feathers have been sterilized. You will also want to look for a comforter with a natural cotton or silk cover that has a high thread count. This will insure the feathers will not poke through the duvet as time goes on. A thread count of 300 or more per square inch is acceptable. Another thing to look for is baffled or boxed construction. This means that the comforter is sewn so that it is sectioned into squares. This prevents the down from shifting too much, which can make for an uneven comforter; warm in one area and cold in the other. There are other things to look for such as fill power, which can be between 500 to 600, and the ounce weight. A 40 ounce weight comforter would be suitable for year-round use while a 55 to 60 ounce weight comforter would be considered winter weight. My comforter is 42 ounce and is warm enough for year-round use. I have never needed to add extra covers about my feet which otherwise tend to get cold. I guarantee it will be one of your better investments towards a quality night's sleep.

If your feet still tend to be chilled at night you might opt for cashmere socks to wear to bed. Like the down comforter, they have their own softness and "loft," trapping warm air pockets between your skin and the material. They are soft enough to not irritate the sensitive skin of diabetic and fibromyalgia patients. To date I know of only one company that can custom-make cashmere socks for such medical applications. *Esterphanie St. Juste* of NYC fills such orders through www.CashmereSocks.com or call (212) 724-6331. This company will take your measurements and make custom cashmere socks to order no matter what your medical condition. They are of excellent quality and made of some of the finest cashmere found anywhere.

The second prerequisite for a rejuvenating night's rest would be the proper mattress. We spend close to one-third of our lives in bed or asleep. No wonder people with sleep disorders will often suffer from depression, fatigue and disorientation after not just weeks but months of poor quality sleep. I have used numerous pads in an attempt to place a layer of cushioning between the mattress and myself. I have used goose down mattress toppers as well as egg crate foam pads with limited success. I even purchased a foam mattress pad that was supposed to have "memory." That was really quite helpful overall and was an improvement over the other pads that I have tried. However, after about a year of use it seemed to have developed Alzheimer's and lost its memory! It no longer responded to the curves and sways of my body. You see, it is these contacts with the mattress that can cause pressure points. You find yourself tossing and turning half the night because circulation diminishes while pressure increases causing discomfort.

What I finally found that worked exceedingly well was a very carefully made densely formed visco-elastic mattress by Tempur-Pedic®. I purchased one of their pillows about a year ago after being in a rear-end accident that left me with constant neck and shoulder pain. It had to be the heaviest pillow I ever felt, yet form follows function here. The visco-elastic foam was first engineered for astronauts, allowing them to comfortably sustain the high pressure and G-forces present at takeoff. Let me say that it works quite well on Earth too. Within a few minutes the heat of your head and weight molds its own unique shape into the pillow. Rather than forcing against you, the pillow supports your neck and spine, providing natural alignment. I have never needed another pillow. Another bonus is the fact that due to the memory molding capacity of the visco-elastic foam, you are not forcing extra wrinkles into your face and neck while sleeping. Do you believe that some beauty books suggest that you sleep on your back to avoid just this scenario? Personally, I think that is just a bit over the top when it comes to vanity. Still, why not purchase a product that can help prevent the problem in the first place?

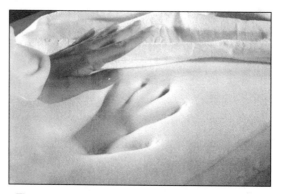

The visco-elastic material supports the spine & joints.

Since the Tempur-Pedic® pillow was so restful, I decided to try their mattress that was on display at a store in a mall near my home. Resting on that mattress, even with people milling about and the store lights on, had to be one of the most relaxing experiences I can recall. Once again, just like the pillow, my body began to sink down as it began to accommodate yet support my unique curves and bony prominences. After sleeping on it for just one night after it arrived in my home, that nagging backache that I have had since my car accident was gone the next morning! After quickly and easily falling asleep, I woke up several hours later in the exact same position. I had not tossed or turned in all that time.

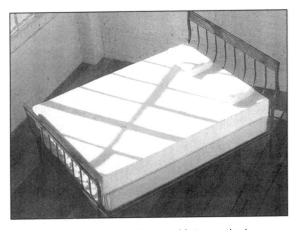

Tempur-Pedic® mattress molds to your body.

Most of us change position between 20 to 30 times per night. Now tell me… with all of that flopping about, however are you supposed to get a restful night's sleep? This was no fluke either. I had to do a book signing where I was required to stay overnight on a different mattress that was lovely and new. I hardly slept, and when I woke up, my back was killing me. I went home and slept again on the Tempur-Pedic® and the next morning, once again, no backache. Perhaps I have been spoiled? Whatever the case, the quality of sleep that I get now from having the proper, supportive mattress is incomparable. Sometimes I used to need a nap in the afternoon just to keep going. No more! The quality of sleep I get at night now has me more energetic and clearer thinking than I can remember being in a long time. My productivity is up and I even have a bit of extra energy to skate and swim three times per week. Amazing.

You can see there are many things that can be done to enhance that marvelous one-third of your life that you spend asleep. A good night's rest cannot be underestimated for its ability to renew and detoxify the body. Still, you must give your body the best possible tools to work with to accomplish what should be considered a minor nightly miracle. To learn more about the Tempur-Pedic® Sleep System call 888-664-2036 or visit on-line at: www.tempurpedic.com.

Chapter 6

GET MOVING TO
GET IN SHAPE

Biking: Good for the Heart & Joints

I f you suffer from painful arthritis, perhaps the last thing
you want to think about is exercise. Certain exercises,
however, are hard on even healthy joints and should
be avoided. They include high impact aerobics, running
and jogging, particularly on hard pavements and surfaces.
The amount of pressure placed on your knees, for example, is increased sevenfold per square inch with each
pounding step. This works to wear away the supportive
cartilage that cushions the ends of the joints. This process
occurs naturally as we age but is accelerated by such activities as just described. It is also aggravated from being
slightly overweight.

Some may feel that this is a "Catch 22" situation. In order to maintain joint mobility and ideal weight, we know
we must exercise, but how? One would most certainly not
want to exacerbate their condition and let's face it; it's really painful making the effort!

There are a few ways around this problem that will
allow you to get the cardiovascular conditioning and circulation of aerobic exercise and at the same time spare

your poor joints.

One form of exercise that is highly recommended is bicycling. The most efficient use of energy for motion known to man, there is practically no stress to the joints of the hips, knees and ankles, target areas for wear and deterioration. Indoor cycling, or "spinning," has become a hot attraction at many posh gyms across the country and offers an alternative to cycling in inclement weather. All terrain bikes are also now very popular because they offer large tires, a comfortable seat and even shocks similar to what you would find on a car. All of these features cushion your ride and prevent your bones from being jarred. With gas prices as high as they are today, you may want to get out your bike and begin saving some money on short trips around town.

To address the problem of joint deterioration, you may also wish to try glucosamine sulfate, a dietary supplement to help rebuild and repair worn cartilage.

Glucosamine (sulfate), an "amino-sugar," is involved in the formation of tendons, bones, ligaments and even heart valves. When combined with a sulfur component, it is then called glucosamine sulfate. Supplementing with glucosamine can also help bursitis, osteoporosis and tendonitis. This is because it is not like other forms of sugar in the body. As an amino sugar, it is used more like amino acids. This means that glucosamine is incorporated into living tissue, rather than being burned as glucose for energy.

Biking is a great way to start on the road to heart health and fitness without doing damage to your joints. You set the pace and build up your endurance slowly as your heart and lungs become conditioned to the increased exercise. As with any exercise program, check with your doctor before starting, especially if you have not exercised in some time.

Skating: Just What the Doctor Ordered

Can you remember, as I can remember, the very first time you put on a pair of skates? No matter if they were the clanking metal types that clipped onto your sneakers or the not so sharp ice skates you found in the basement. That ultimate feeling of freedom and near flight was intoxicating! There's one thing for sure. There is absolutely no reason why you cannot relive the same joy that you felt in your youth.

Like biking, skating offers little or no stress on the joints. You can get an excellent cardiovascular workout by skating for only one hour three times a week. Here is where the real bonus comes in for us women. Doing swizzles, or small stroking movements with the feet, helps tone both the inner and outer thighs as well as the buttocks and calves. There is nothing better than aerobic exercise out-of-doors where there is plenty of free oxygen to enjoy. This is what makes skating an exercise that you can stick with over time. Think about it. No classes at the gym to schedule, no repetitious lifting. Strap on your skates and pick the scenery you would like to the see for the day. You can burn up to 400 calories an hour skating and you will increase your metabolism for up to 48 hours after you stop.

Whether you are comfortable on "quad" skates, used mostly in the roller rink, or ice skates there is no reason why you should give up thoughts of using them again. I can remember my father buying me my first pair of roller rink skates. I was 15 and was just starting to go out on dates at the roller rink and movies. They were the traditional four-wheel (quad) skates with a high white leather boot. They also had a toe stop on the front with hard wheels that housed speedy ball bearings. Do you know that I still have them and they still fit? I continued to skate with them up until 1992 when I was ready for a radical change. Enter in-line skates. I purchased my first pair of

Rollerblades® (yes, the brand name), specifically their T R S Lightnings. I was instantly able to skate backwards, which was a skill that I never mastered on the quads. Not only that, but the urethane wheels were much softer and gripped better than my old skates. They were actually quite comfortable from the first day out. Since my conversion in 1992, I have never gone back to skating with quads. Rollerblade® first offered their in-line skate to the market in 1980.

You might be thinking that skating on in-line skates is much more difficult than on quads. The only difficulty I had in changing over was negotiating the slightly longer wheelbase of the in-line skate, which includes a back brake. You have to be aware of the extra length when doing crossovers. Otherwise the brake can get in the way and cause you to fall during this maneuver. Another challenge is that in order to engage the brake you have to extend your leg in front of you while bending your other knee. You are in effect pushing your heel out in front of you, which is in and of itself a very unnatural position. Some more advanced models of in-line skates have heel cuffs that will engage the brake simply by leaning back on it. Unfortunately these more sophisticated braking systems are often found on the off-road, extreme skating models such as the Rollerblade® Coyote. Just in case you are interested, these babies have 6-inch air filled wheels and drum brakes! The bearings are rain-sealed so you can pretty much slosh through the snow and mud to your heart's content if you are so inclined. (Yes, I own a pair of Coyotes.)

If you have ever ice-skated, you might find in-line skating to be quite familiar. On quad skates you have four edges to manage while the in-line skates only have two. There are two edges on an ice skate also. Corresponding to in-line skates you have both an inside and outside edge. If you have had any success or experience ice skating, you might wish to give in-line skating a try. There are also benefits of learning to in-line skate as opposed to quad skating. For one thing, as previously mentioned, it is very similar to ice skating. Many figure skaters will keep on top of their form during the off-season by simply doing a little recreational roller-blading. You can also practice and improve your skiing technique, such as slaloms and downhill turns, using in-line skates. The muscles that you engage for all of these activities are virtually the same. Each time that you practice the motion, your muscle's memory of how to execute these maneuvers becomes more finely tuned. This is what is known as cross training. You are using different equipment but effecting the same goals of balance and coordination.

Still a little leery? Consider only skating in a controlled environment such as a hockey, ice or roller rink. There is also some very high tech protection equipment available apart from the usual knee and elbow pads, wrist guards and helmets. If you have not skated for a long time you might need to invest in new pair of skates that fit properly. Some skates are unisex while others are lasted to fit the female anatomy. Companies such as Rollerblade® and K2® have a long reputation of respecting the uniqueness of the female foot and leg. For one thing we tend to have narrower heels and higher insteps than our male counterparts. Also, a woman's calve is naturally shorter than a man's. The boot cuff designed for a man's foot can actually cut into the back of a woman's leg resulting in chaffing and discomfort.

In order to counteract the problems of uncomfortable boots, especially when they are new, K2® first addressed this by developing and patenting a soft boot design. However, a lawsuit against Salomon, a rival skate company, for patent infringement by inline skate manufacturer K2® was settled out of court, with Salomon agreeing to discontinue sales of its TR series in the United States. Salomon had to pull their skates off the shelves in the Unites States and was supposed to have come up with a new skate design in 2001. In the meantime, skating enthusiasts have moved on to a new top-rated skate. Not surprisingly, they have turned to the K2® and 2001 was a banner year in sales for them.

Others have tried to copy K2® but in my opinion, stick with the originator! K2's® soft boot technology closely resembles an athletic shoe or sneaker. Most even have breathable vents to allow for the circulation of air, which keeps the boot cooler and drier. The soft boot is supported by an exo-skeleton, or hard cuff, surrounding it. These are extraordinarily comfortable to wear but need to be strapped up and tightened quite well to give you the support needed. Keep in mind that most in-line skates on the market today are either recreational or fitness skates. This means that the wheels are anywhere from 78 to 80 mm in size. They are well suited for roadwork and traveling in a straight-line mile after mile. However, if you want a skate that will respond to more intricate footwork and maneuvering, you will need a smaller wheel of approximately 70 to 76 mm. Aggressive skates used for street or "vert" skating on ramps have these smaller wheels, but don't expect a stroll through the park in them!

I foolishly tried a pair of Salomon aggressive skates, which nearly landed me on my face. The wheels were extremely sticky with little or no roll out. I am an intermediate to advanced skater but I did nothing but trip and stumble. Some street skaters say that Salomon's "grind slow," so maybe that is just inherent to the brand. In addition to a smaller wheel size, you will need to see if the model skate you wish to purchase has a rockered frame. This allows you to either lengthen or shorten the wheelbase by moving the wheels closer together or further apart on the frame. You can also raise the rear and front wheels on the frame, which allows you to turn and corner more easily.

If you are ready for the next level in skating, consider this. While recreational skating is wonderful, many of us may have a need for artistic expression as well. Figure skating is perhaps the epitome of this art form. However, we may not always have access to an ice rink. Enter the PIC® Skate! The PIC® skate was invented by John Petell and Nick Perna of Harmony Sports. This skate offers a high quality leather reinforced ice skating boot as its foundation. This is serious sports equipment and not to be confused with the boots that are attached to most in-line skates. No, indeed. This is the same type of boot that world class figure skaters depend on to execute their spins, jumps and precision footwork. The frame is of an aluminum alloy that is both lightweight and strong. The main feature of the PIC® frame is the fact that the wheels are rockered. As mentioned before, this allows for intricate turns and twists, just as if you are on the ice. The next great innovation of this skate is the fact that it has the toe stop on the front of the frame. This makes the skate easier to stop and maybe more familiar to those who grew up with quad skates which likewise had a toe stop. The result is a more secure feeling of control and braking ability when you need it most. The toe stop, or pick, on the front of the PIC® Skate acts just like the toe pick on an ice skate. Using the same pick, you can execute jumps and spins that before were only possible on ice skates. Many people who have used in-line skates in the past have left them behind for the PIC® Skate. This may be because after months of road work in a straight-line mile after mile, the soul yearns for a bit more artistic expression.

Getting In Gear

Now that you have a few skate types in mind, no matter what form of skating you choose you are going to need protective gear. Contrary to popular belief, even ice skaters wear protective padding. It is just not as visible as the traditional black wrist, knee and elbow pads we are accustomed to seeing on in-line skaters. One company makes such undetectable protective padding that you really need to look twice to even notice it. When you bring home your new pair of skates, no matter how comfortable they were in the store, make sure you also get the following products to help the break-in period pass as smoothly and pain free as possible:

Clear Clouds™, manufactured by Skating Safe, Inc. (1-888-299-2553 or visit www.SkatingSafe.com) are soothing gel pads and real life savers. Put in your sock as a cushion between your skin and your new boot, but be prepared to be amazed. You will immediately find that you can tighten your boot snugly, thus increasing control and accuracy in your skating. All while protecting the delicate skin from the chaffing edges of a new boot that has not had the time to soften and conform to the contours of your foot and leg. Clear Clouds™ are made of medical grade gel and are odor and bacteria resistant. They can be worn directly against the skin under tights or socks. They make ankle wraps, ankle disks, lace bite pads and knee and hip protectors of the same resilient material. In my opinion, they are the only way to break in a brand new pair of skates.

API Hockey® makes lace bite pads that seem to do what the Clear Clouds™ do. They are made of foam and offer a bit more bulk than the other product although they are used in a similar fashion.

Foot Menders® (www.gordonshoes.com or call 412-587-1754) combines the soothing gel found in Clear Clouds™ with a compression bandage. The gel disc is held in place because it is attached to the bandage itself. My favorite is the ankle sleeve. It is a tubular piece that looks much like a section cut out of pantyhose. You simply slip the sleeve over your foot and ankle, leaving the toes exposed. This is great for general boot cuff and ankle discomfort that is common when breaking in new skates. If you need more specific protection over the ankle bone, or malleolus, Foot Menders® also makes an ankle sleeve with the gel disc built right in.

Many different manufacturers make *wrist guards and*

knee and elbow pads. Salomon®, K2® and Rollerblade® are all good brands. One company, Ultrawheels®, makes knee and elbow pads to fit the shape of a woman's knee-caps and elbows. Ultrawheels® has them labeled under Women's Specific Design. They are less bulky than many of the other brands and are lined with Cool-Max® material and gel padded. They are sleeker and give you a more feminine silhouette. Sometimes that is important when you are out sweating and breathing heavy on the road, which will happen! Nonetheless, this is essential protective equipment.

If you plan to do more of your skating in a controlled environment such as a skating rink, you might be able to simply use the wrist guards. This is because when you fall your natural reflex is to brace yourself with your arms. If you fall with enough force, you could break your wrists. For the same reason depending on where you plan to skate, you may need a helmet also. If you are skating outdoors on any type of pavement, always use a helmet.

Arch Support, or Orthotics, can be added to any skate to improve both fit and performance. In fact, many professional skaters have their custom boots fitted with just these features. Some skating mavens insist that you should not put anything inside your skate but your foot. This of course is poor advice. One problem that is often seen with new skates is extreme pain in the right foot or both feet after only skating a short period time. If the pain radiates from the bottom of your foot or the arch area, more than likely you need a little added support there. Many skaters develop flat feet, which are painfully fallen arches. You can purchase arch supports that are similar to what are used in athletic shoes. Try picking up pencils with your toes. This curling exercise helps to redefine the arch of the foot. If you do not have time for this exercise, simply add a pair of arch supports.

Lights are not only cool but also essential for night time visibility. Spaghetti Lites™, available from

AimDiscount.com at www.aimdiscount.com/CBlite.html can be used on your skates, helmet and even your body. They can even be wrapped around your waist or jacket for extra visibility, which is really important if you plan to do nighttime skating as I do. With the Spaghetti Lites,™ you simply stick them onto your skate boot or frame and they glow a beautiful neon color that is hard to miss (that's the point, right?)

Bone Up On The Sport

There is much to know about skating even though you may feel that you have learned everything as a child. Not so. In order to skate with confidence, balance and precision you will need to learn about your equipment and how it works. Quad skates have not really changed much over the years, so if you are comfortable with this style of skating, by all means continue. However, as you may well know these types of skates can only be used in a roller rink setting. This fact may limit the amount of time and opportunity you have to use your skates. Basically the same holds true for ice skates unless you live in a very cold climate where ice ponds abound. If you choose in-line skates, you can skate in both the rink and outside. So while the choice is yours, you should invest a little time getting to know how to use your new equipment.

There are several videotapes as well as books that can assist you in learning and developing proper skating technique. One such book written by Liz Miller gets you started with the basics. *Get Rolling* is full of pictures, diagrams and information that will help you improve your skating technique. I especially like the way the material is broken down so that when you combine all the elements you end up with a successful execution of the maneuver. Ms. Miller also has a second book, *Advanced In-line Skating,* which goes beyond the beginners' edition.

If you are interested in artistic skating with your in-line skates you need to get *How to Jump & Spin on In-*

line Skates by Jo Ann Schneider Farris. This book tells you everything you need to know regarding ice skating techniques on in-line skates, particularly utilizing the PIC® Skate frame. One of this book's success stories actually began to do jumps and spins at age 44 after reading the book! So never think it's too late. Just be sure to strap on those Clear Clouds ™ hip protectors first!

The Best Skates For Women

Women today want it all and can most certainly have it. Who says exercise has to be boring, repetitive and difficult? Why not exercise AND express yourself artistically at the same time? For this reason, my PIC® Skates are my utmost favorites. I have the Pro 700 model because not only are they absolutely beautiful, but the boot will hold up through jumps and spins. The very first minute I tried them on, I was able to skate backwards with ease and speed. I was even able to do a pivot! These skates are truly a miracle on wheels. The toe pick allows you to stop quickly and even jump. The rockered frame makes turns so easy. Best of all they are suitable for beginners.

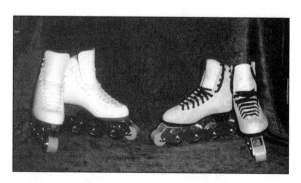

Harmony Sport's PIC® Skates

I like to customize my skates to make them a little "cooler," at least for my tastes. I have changed the wheels from a 70 mm to a 72 mm Hyper® Superlite Wheel with a durometer, or hardness, of 78A. I also installed ABEC 7 bearings in these slightly larger wheels for a longer roll out. That means with one push, you glide a little further. Just remember, big wheels allow you to go faster while smaller wheels give you more control for turns and spins. The PIC® Skates use Canadian-made GAM boots, which are some of the best-made leather skating boots in the world. They support you like nothing else and are heat-moldable for instant fit and comfort. The only other thing I added was a pair of Dr. Scholl's® gel pads. PIC® Skates are absolutely phenomenal and the best skate of any kind I have ever owned.

My favorite inline skates are my K2® Slip Fit Cadence and Syncro (2002 recreational model) and Rollerblade's® 2002 Lightning 05 and Core 07. All are lasted for a woman's foot; therefore, the boot is soft and constructed much like an athletic shoe. The K2® frames have rockering ability although not to the degree the PIC® Skates have. Still they are fun and suitable for outdoor recreational use or even in the rink...your choice. The wheels are a 78A in hardness, which means they are softer and grip better than a harder wheel of 80 or 82A. They also absorb more of the bumps and shocks of the road. K2 uses Twin Cam ABEC 5 bearings that have virtually no break-in time and are excellent quality. I chose to install BSB speed bearings in my K2® Cadence skates but there is little difference between those and the Twin Cam ABEC 5 bearings they came with since they were so smooth right out of the box.

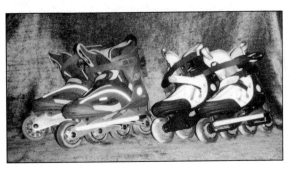

K2's® 2002 Cadence & Syncro models.

You should check the wheels before buying to make sure all of the wheels rotate freely. Even if they don't right away, after a couple of trips out, they should loosen up. However, make sure to keep an eye on the situation. Sticky or slow bearings mean you have to work harder to overcome the extra friction they are causing. Your roll-out should be smooth and even from all wheels. The K2s® especially are VERY light and comfortable the first day you try them on. While you cannot execute as many ice skating maneuvers with them as you could with the PIC® Skate, you can still obtain more precision in your skating due to the rockered frame. I am always modifying my equipment, so I took off the brake. I can do a C and a T stop pretty well so skating without a back brake isn't all that scary. I also only skate in controlled environments. This means an outdoor hockey rink or indoor roller rink. I don't like surprises and skating in city traffic could leave you surprisingly dead!

Skating in a safe location allows you to focus more on your technique and skills without worrying if the neighbor's pit bull got out again or if that pebble you didn't notice is going to send you for a tumble.

Rollerblade® has a new line of their Lightning Series that includes the Lightning 05. It has a slightly lower cuff but still provides support and is the ultimate in the "get you sweaty" fitness skate. This seems to be the new wave and the fastest growing segment of inline skating as people are leaving the gym and seeking cardiovascular toning and fitness out of doors. The Lightning 05's 82 mm wheels are super-light Rollerblade® manufactured wheels with even lighter and faster microbearings that make these skates eerily similar to 5 wheel speed skates but with a more secure ride in mind. Rollerblade,® ever the innovator, decided to keep the speed laces that in my opinion provide a much better fit. The better your movements transfer to your equipment, the better your skating will be. The new generation of Rollerblades® is on the cutting edge of hybrid skates, which combine the best features from other styles and models with all the bells and whistles. It seems no detail was overlooked in making these skates comfortable and easy fitting from the beginning. The result is a skate with its own personality and attitude that gives you limitless possibilities.

A skate that I did not have very much success with is the Ultrawheels® Bioflex 2001 FX7L whose frame actually flexes with each stride and returns to its original position by way of a spring. There is a lot of technology built into these skates but I am not sure how it translates onto the road. I found the fit of the Ultrawheels® to be less comfortable than the K-2's®; however, I experienced this only over the anklebones. This is where gel ankle pads such as the Clear Clouds™ will be most helpful. They can allow you a custom fit from the very first time you try on new skates.

The foot bed on the Ultrawheels® was also a bit wide, especially for a woman's foot. I have normal, everyday feet. Not "narrow triple A" or "extra wide" and these skates were quite loose at the toe and ball of the foot. Ultrawheel's® 2002 model of the Bioflex FX7L sports a more maneuverable 76 mm wheel with ABEC 7 bearings. The style is also impressive.

Another skate that I would not recommend is Salomon's® XTR-Quattros, which I found to be very similar to the fit and feel of the Ultrawheels.® Like the Ultrawheels,® they are manufactured in Thailand. Also like the Ultrawheels,® the fit of the boot seems to be more suited for a wider foot. While the Salomon® Quattros did not exactly hurt my ankles, as did the Ultrawheels,® they did hurt my arches horribly after having them on for only a few minutes. Also, the fit of the cuff was boxy and uncomfortable. If you are going to learn and continue to skate properly, fit is everything!

Some skate salesmen have said that you either have a K2® foot or a Salomon foot. K2s® are narrower, tapered and fit like a glove. K2® has put a lot of technology into their Fit-Logic system, which others have tried and failed to duplicate. Salomon's® fit perhaps would be better suited for someone with extra-wide feet, but even with that the foot bed is boxy and uncomfortable, at least for my feet. Since I consider my foot to be about average for a female, I would strongly suggest getting the K2s® for a perfect fit every time.

Inspiration From Women Just Like Us

Paula Soloby and Nancy Bronisevsky are regular American girls just like us. The only difference is that they bloomed somewhat later in life when it comes to entering the sport of artistic skating. Sports of any kind for women over the age of 30 are generally not encouraged. Fear and risk of injury or simply feeling that we are past our competitive prime may hinder many of us from even trying. To this end, Soloby and Bronisevsky are Mavericks in their field. They have combined their need for exercise and partici-pating in a sport usually associated with children. Rather than sit on the sidelines while their children skate, they got out there with them and found enjoyment for them-selves.

For example, Paula began skating after her son went off to college. She had always walked to stay in shape but became bored of the monotony of that routine. She then visited a local roller skating rink, put on a pair of rentals and began to enjoy the music. Her experience as a competitive disco dancer connected with her affinity for rhythm. Soon after she began taking private lessons and advanced to the competitive level after only a year. She is now regional champion in solo dance and figures and is state champion in dance. Not bad!

Nancy began by bringing her three daughters to the rink for fun but soon found that she enjoyed the activity along with them. So her daughters began to take lessons and she soon followed with adult lessons. Nancy lost weight and firmed up considerably while increasing her cardiovascular capacity. To her surprise she won third place in dance and third in figures her first time competing. She looks great and has a lot more energy while participating in an activity that simply does not feel like exercise. Nancy says that she really looks forward to her skating sessions. "I wake up saying, oh great, it's Tuesday! I'll be skating today!" When was the last time you felt that level of enthusiasm for exercise? Career wise, Nancy has gotten an unexpected boost. She is now training to be a counselor for Weight Watchers®!

Not quite ready for such a leap? Well, I have found group lessons for beginners to be far less intimidating. I have attended classes with my 8-year-old and her "little" friends! Who cares? We have a professional skating coach, Carey Elder of Jackson Rollermagic, who has been skating since he was 10 and has coached both ice and roller-skating. He has also won numerous skating championships and choreographed a fox trot now named for him. "I've seen mothers bring their children for lessons and end up taking lessons themselves." Elder relates. Not a bad idea since you should be well acquainted with how to stop and even fall safely.

Here you have artistic expression, cardiovascular conditioning, muscle toning and lots of laughs while you're at it. The key is to engage in an activity that you can stick with over time. You are also more apt to stay with a program where you can learn and incorporate new techniques. This in and of itself is a great confidence builder. You will find yourself looking forward to the next opportunity to try something new in your skating. Stretching the limits of your physical abilities is very gratifying. You needn't have a gym membership in order to get exercise, either. Many parks are now building roller hockey rinks that are often empty early in the morning. Rather than taking a jog in the park, how about taking a glide instead? Much less stress on the joints and twice the enjoyment!

Chapter 7

R E F R E S H – R E N E W

Nothing, and I mean nothing, is better after a full workout than to be able to relax in a warm bath. Studies indicate that activities such as massage and warm soaks help the brain to release endorphins, or "feel good" hormones, which are related to opiates. They allow us to relax and fully enjoy the pleasure signals our bodies are receiving. After exercise your muscles have built up lactic acid which, if not removed, can cause cramping and those nighttime Charlie horses that are known to disturb anyone's sleep. A warm dip or immersion helps improve circulation, thus facilitating the removal of lactic acid from muscles.

High-end spas all over the world are capitalizing on this simple pleasure. However, with a little preparation, innovation and inspiration you can easily duplicate these wonderful treatments for pennies without leaving the comfort of your own home. The ingredients can be purchased at your local supermarket and health food store. Ready? Following are a few exotic pleasures that I know you will enjoy.

Recipes for the Body & Bath

Reprinted with permission from *How Flowers Heal* by Marie Anakee Miczak, Writer's Club Press.

* * *

Using essential oils and fresh flowers for body care and bath items is a real treat and can be quite simple. Unless noted otherwise most of the items should be refrigerated and kept for no longer than a week. The longer the product sits, the more likely the active ingredients will dissipate and the overall concoction will become less effective. Remember to use the freshest ingredients possible and real Aromatherapy-grade essential oils.

Vanilla Rose Body Oil

> 4 tablespoons olive oil
>
> 4 tablespoons sweet almond oil
>
> 1 teaspoon pure vanilla extract
>
> 1 cup fresh or ½ cup dried rose petals
>
> 5 drops rose essential oil (optional)

Place oils and rose petals in a clean glass bottle. Let stand in your refrigerator for one week. After that period of time, strain off plant material and add vanilla and essential oil. Mix well before using, as the vanilla may tend to separate. If you like, you can use essential oil of vanilla.

Basic Massage Oil

> ¼ cup sweet almond oil
>
> 2 tablespoons olive oil
>
> ½ teaspoon cocoa butter (optional)

Combine and heat ingredients until warm. Add either essential oil or plant matter of choice. You can add up to 15 drops of pure essential oil or 2 tablespoons of dried or fresh leaves, petals, etc. If using the latter, let the plant material steep in hot oil for 5 to 10 minutes, depending on desired strength. Strain oil through a sieve and place in a clean, sterilized bottle. Store in the refrigerator between uses. The blends for perfumes may be used to scent the massage oil or single notes of essential oils such as lavender, rose, geranium, etc. You will find these particular massage oils perfect for after-bath moisturizing.

Honey Rose Body Oil

    4 tablespoons sweet almond oil

    1 teaspoon corn oil

    2 tablespoons olive oil

    ½ teaspoon natural honey

    5 drops essential oil of rose

    1 to 2 teaspoons vitamin E oil

    1 teaspoon powdered rose petal (optional)

To prepare powdered rose petal, first dry the petals as you would for use in potpourri. Using a small coffee grinder or mortar and pestle, pulverize them into a fine powder. Store in a tin container in a cool, dark place until ready to use. Discard if any mold appears.

Mix all ingredients together and heat for a couple of seconds in the microwave to help the ingredients blend together. Store in the refrigerator between uses. This formula works especially well to help soften rough patches of skin such as on the elbows and knees. Apply as often as you like.

The vitamin E and honey will help act as natural preservatives; therefore this body oil will have a longer shelf life. Discard if any signs of rancidity form, which can be detected by a strong odor not related to the aromatic floral extractions.

Violet All Over Body Silk

    6 tablespoons olive oil

    1 teaspoon corn oil

    ¼ teaspoon natural honey

    ¼ teaspoon natural beeswax

    ¼ cup dried or ½-cup fresh violet flowers and leaves

Heat the first four ingredients in a small pot or sauce pan. When beeswax has melted and oil is hot add the dried or fresh violet. Stir constantly with a metal spoon. The fresh plant material may seem like too much at first but once it gets heated and starts to absorb the oil, it will wilt down. Turn the heat off, cover the pot and let steep for 20 to 30 minutes. Strain off the plant material and place in a clean, sterilized glass jar. Plastic will also do. Keep refrigerated in between uses. The beeswax will help the oils and honey solidify. If you would like a harder salve, add more beeswax. If you can find it, a few drops of violet essential oil is a great addition.

Floral Body Drenchers

Floral waters are quite simple to make and use as body mists. Simply place dried or fresh flowers of choice in 2 to 4 cups spring water. Bring water to a boil and then turn heat down and let simmer for 5 minutes. Turn the heat completely off and cover. Let steep for 10 to 20 minutes. The longer it sits in the water, the stronger the scent and medicinal qualities will become. Once finished steeping, strain through a sieve if you don't mind some remaining plant matter or with a paper coffee filter. Place in a clean, sterilized glass container and store in the refrigerator.

    You can also use a method of making "sun teas" to make your floral waters. Add flowers and essential oil to water in a clear glass jar or bottle. Place in a sunny windowsill or area on the porch/deck. This method can take anywhere from one to seven days depending on the plant(s) being used. To apply, either use an air pump spray bottle to mist yourself frequently or use it as an all-over body splash right after a shower. Both ways are quite refreshing. The preparation and use of floral waters dates back to ancient Egypt, Greek and Roman eras. Depending on the type of flower you choose, these waters can be quite beneficial to the healing of skin disorders such as acne, psoriases, eczema, etc. Pour a cup or two into your next bath for an added treat or mix in a few teaspoons of dried clay powder to make a wonderful mask.

The various uses for these floral waters are enormous!

Natural Lavender Bath Powder

½ cup cornstarch

½ cup rice flour

¼ cup dried lavender flowers (ground or pulverized)

3 drops lavender essential oil

Grind the lavender to a fine powder consistency. Add it to the flour and cornstarch. Mix well. Add a few drops of essential oil such as benzoin to act as a natural preservative. Store in a tin or plastic container and let cure for one week in the refrigerator. Being that this is made from natural ingredients, it is best to store it in the refrigerator to prolong the shelf life. Perfect for after-bath-dusting in the evening since this recipe has the added bonus of assisting a good nights sleep. Once again you can use this same recipe with any of the perfume recipes to develop your own personal scent collection.

Silky Ylang Ylang Powder

1½ cup cornstarch

5 drops ylang ylang essential oil

1 teaspoon sweet almond oil or any extremely light oil such as jojoba

Mix all ingredients together using a blender or a sealed plastic bag. Both ways will provide equal results. Empty into a clean container and let cure 5 to 7 days so that the scent mingles with the cornstarch. If you like, you can add a few teaspoons of orrisroot powder to act as a natural preservative. This is an excellent recipe for people with dry skin. The added oil will help moisturize and calm the skin. Great for use in the morning or anytime.

Geranium Deodorant Powder

> 1 cup cornstarch
>
> 2 tablespoons baking powder
>
> 1 teaspoon orrisroot (optional)
>
> 5 to 10 drops geranium essential oil

Mix all ingredients well in a blender or use a sealed plastic bag. Empty into a clean container and let cure for 5 to 7 days. Store in the refrigerator to help keep it fresh. Use a large powdered sugar shaker to dispense, if you like. It is very gentle yet very effective. Geranium essential oil is a great deodorant along with the baking soda. You can sprinkle this in your shoes and on your bedding as well. It is not simply covering the odor with a perfume but neutralizing it, therefore it is important that you use a quality geranium essential oil and not a fragrance oil, which is pure synthetic scent.

Variation:

Peppermint Foot Powder

Instead of the geranium essential oil add peppermint and ground peppermint leaves, which are easily made in a small coffee grinder. Mix everything well and let cure for a week. This works well when rubbed on the ankles and soles of the feet to help deodorize. You may also sprinkle it anywhere that requires the energizing scent of real peppermint!

Petal Soaps

Making your own floral soaps is simple when you use pre-made soap and dried flowers.

Fill a small pot with cold water and bring it to a fast simmer. Place glycerin soap, which has been cubed into small chunks, inside a plastic zip lock bag and close the top. Place this bag into another self-closing plastic bag and tie it closed. Place bag in simmering water and dip and move it around until the soap has melted. As soon as it has, remove the bag from the water and wipe off the outside of the bag well. Just like with melting chocolate, getting water into the soap will ruin it.

Take a small tea box and line it with tin foil. Spray a little cooking oil inside if you like. If you do not want to use a tea box you can buy special molds made for soaps from most craft stores or places that sell Aromatherapy products. Immediately pour half of your soap into the lined tea box. Sprinkle flower petals of your choice onto the layer of soap. If they are large, whole flower heads take a toothpick and push them down into the soap layer. Pour the remaining hot, melted soap over the first layer and store the box in a well ventilated, dry area. The heat in the soap will help draw out the medicinal and aromatic attributes of the herbs you added.

Essential oils can also be added to your soap by adding the oil to the bag containing the glycerin soap chunks. The essential oils are then absorbed into the hot soap. Use Aromatherapy or perfume blending charts to determine which combinations work best.

After your soap has cooled completely, take a warm knife with a little oil on it and slice your large block of floral soap into bars. Wrap the bars tightly in tissue paper and let them cure for up to one week.

Variation:

Mosaic Petal Soaps

To make interesting mosaic soaps, simply take pre-made floral white soaps that are too small to be used anymore and cut them into small cubes or chunks. Do not use glycerin soaps because they will melt and not provide the same effect. A creamy white soap is recommended. Pour some melted glycerin soap into the bottom of the lined tea box. Add the cubed white or Castille soap and flower petals. Use a toothpick to push them down. Pour more glycerin soap over the top. Prepare as previously described.

Mosaic soaps are wonderful because they are unusual and you can use commercial, non-glycerin soap for the interesting effect. If you want your mosaic soap to be deep cleansing, use oatmeal soap cubes. For softening your skin, use lavender soap cubes.

Rose Bath Oil

½ cup vegetable or sweet almond oil

20 drops rose essential oil

¼ cup fresh or dried rose petals

¼ teaspoon natural, pure honey (optional)

Combine all ingredients into an open mouth glass bottle. Allow it to sit in your refrigerator for about 1 week. After it has cured, remove the rose petals and store in the refrigerator between uses. To use, add a couple tablespoons to hot bath water and enjoy. Works well on very dry skin conditions and in the wintertime.

Peach Rose Bubble Bath

5 drops peach fragrance oil

10 drops rose essential oil

¼ cup dried rose petals (optional)

1 bar natural glycerin soap

¼ to ½ cup rose water

Melt soap as previously described for making Petal Soaps. Place the rose petals, essential oils and fragrance oils into the bottom of a wide mouth glass jar. Pour in the rose water and then add the hot, melted soap. Place a top on the jar and shake the mixture well. It will thicken as the soap cools. Store in the refrigerator between uses. To use, add a couple of tablespoons under hot running water. May also be used as a delicate body wash.

Recipes for the Complexion & Special Beauty Treatments

There are many traditional recipes that include flowers as their base ingredient for beautifying the complexion and skin. Many ancient cultures believed that creating concoctions containing flowers, which were lovely to look at, would transfer their beauty to the human using it. While this may or may not be true many flowers, especially rose and lavender, can do wondrous things for the skin, including reducing fine lines and clearing up acne. Before trying the following recipes, remember to do a patch test! The skin of the face can be very sensitive, especially when raw botanicals are used.

Age Defying Oil

2 cups fresh calendula flowers

1 cup olive oil

4 teaspoons vitamin E oil

Place flowers in the oil and allow to steep in the refrigerator for a few days. Strain off botanical matter and apply the oil to the whole face, or where lines appear, twice a week.

Rose Milk Complexion Mask

¼ cup whole milk

¼ cup heavy cream (optional)

10 drops essential oil of rose

½ teaspoon vanilla extract (optional)

Combine all ingredients well and apply to the entire face, paying special attention to avoid the eye area, and allow to dry on the face for 15 to 30 minutes. Store any remaining mask in the refrigerator for no longer than a week. This mask can also be applied to other parts of the body such as the shoulders, knees, elbows, etc.

Petal Mask

¼ cup fresh rose petals

1 teaspoon dried lavender or lavender tea

2 drops rose essential oil (optional)

2 drops lavender essential oil (optional)

1 whole egg beaten

1 teaspoon fresh lemon juice or pure lemon extract

1 teaspoon vanilla extract

2 tablespoons dried milk powder

Combine all ingredients in a small bowl and stir for 50 strokes or until completely combined. Allow to rest in the refrigerator for 10 minutes, then spread over the entire face and neck, paying special attention to avoid the eye and mouth area. Leave on for about 15 to 20 minutes, then rinse off with warm water. Apply a moisturizing treatment afterwards.

This mask not only smells heavenly, but will firm the skin wonderfully and really leave it smooth. Some like to use this as a hand treatment as well.

Rose Hip Buttermilk Mask

½ cup crushed rose hips

¼ cup spring water

¼ cup buttermilk

2 tablespoons dried milk powder

2 drops rose essential oil (optional)

Bring the water to a boil and quickly add the rose hips. Turn the heat off immediately. Allow the mixture to steep until the water is cooled. Strain off the rose hips and add buttermilk and milk powder. To achieve a thicker mask, add more milk powder to get the consistency you desire. Apply to the entire face, being sure to avoid the eye area. Allow the mask to remain for up to 30 minutes. Rinse with warm water.

Elder Flower Complexion Elixir

1/2 cup dried elder flower blossoms

1 cup spring water

2 drops lavender essential oil (optional)

Pour the boiling water over the dried elder flowers and allow the mixture to steep until the water is cool. Strain off the plant matter and add lavender oil, if applicable. Place the liquid in a glass bottle with a secure lid and store in the refrigerator between uses. Apply by soaking a washcloth in the elixir and gently applying it to the entire face in a circular pattern.

Chamomile Eye Elixir

1 bag black tea

1/3 cup spring water

4 tablespoons dried chamomile flowers

2 drops essential oil of Roman chamomile

Bring the water to a boil and add the tea and chamomile

flowers. Turn the heat off and allow the tea to steep for 15 minutes or until cool. Strain off the botanical matter and add the essential oil. Place in a glass container and store in the refrigerator between uses. To use, soak a cotton ball in the solution and apply around the eye area, in an inward motion starting from the edge of the eye and working in towards the nose. Leave on for 5 minutes, then rinse off gently with warm water.

Clarifying Oil

 4 tablespoons violet flowers

 4 tablespoons sage

 5 tablespoons almond or jojoba oil

 3 capsules vitamin E oil

 2 drops lavender essential oil (optional)

Combine all of the ingredients. Allow the mixture to steep in the refrigerator for 1 to 2 weeks. Be sure to shake or stir the mixture everyday. Once cured, apply the oil to the skin using a cotton ball. This is very good for clearing-up skin conditions such as minor acne and helping the skin to heal faster, reducing scaring. May also be used on the lips to help stop cold sores from forming.

Rose Facial Moisturizer

 1/3 teaspoon vegetable shortening

 1 teaspoon jojoba or sweet almond oil

 2 teaspoons fresh lemon juice

 5 drops rose essential oil

 1 teaspoon dried rose petals (optional)

Combine all of the ingredients in a small pot or double boiler over low heat. Heat the mixture until liquefied. Remove from heat and pour into a small container. Allow the moisturizer to set in the refrigerator. Apply to the face, paying special attention to dry skin areas.

Floral Facial Gel

 1 teaspoon dried lavender or lavender tea

 4 drops lavender essential oil (optional)

 1/2 cup aloe vera gel

 1 teaspoon chamomile tea

 1 teaspoon calendula tea

Combine all of the ingredients and place in a microwave-safe container. Heat in the microwave for approximately 1 or 2 minutes or until liquefied. Allow to cool slightly. Strain off the plant material if you like. Place in the refrigerator to set completely. Use on the entire face as an evening or morning treatment.

Chapter 8

NATURAL HAIR CARE

Every year women spend billions of dollars on hair care products. Why not? After all, our hair is our crowning glory! Still, you need to be a savvy consumer and realize that there is more hype than reality to these products. Not only that, many commercial hair colorants contain heavy metals such as lead, which is not a good thing to absorb into your scalp. Also, there are allergic reactions associated with the use of many types of hair dyes. Carol Channing, for instance, can no longer use many chemical products on her skin or scalp. Years of bleaching and coloring her hair have left her very sensitive to most chemical additives.

Going gray is a natural part of aging, albeit premature graying is yet another issue. The lighter strands of silver and gray soften the effect around our faces. Think of them as well-earned highlights!

Now you can have your cake and eat it too. The following natural hair color enhancers and treatments add luster to your hair naturally with no chemicals. The botanicals included in these formulations actually strengthen the hair, not weaken it, as do hydrogen peroxide based hair dyes. You owe it to yourself and your hair to do the best for both. Beautiful hair should not come at the sacrifice of your overall health. If you have a favorite natural shampoo, you might wish to amplify its benefits by adding essential oils and botanicals to them. The result will be a super synergy that combines the best that nature has to offer.

Floral Recipes for the Hair

There are many floral botanicals that can nourish and bring life back to stressed out tresses! Essential oils can also be used with great success, especially in commercially bought products, since only a few drops are needed to enhance the product. Rosemary and chamomile are two of the most useful botanicals for the scalp and hair and may be used in either herbal or essential oil form.

Natural Chamomile Shampoo

- ½ cup soapwort (sweet William)
- ¼ cup chamomile flowers
- 1 teaspoon commercial, non-scented shampoo (optional)
- 2 drops chamomile essential oil (optional)
- 2 cups spring or rain water

Combine the soapweed, chamomile and shampoo. Pour boiling water over the mixture until it turns an amber color. Keep it refrigerated between uses. Since it contains less detergent than what you are probably used to with commercial products, you may need to leave the mixture on your hair for up to 15 minutes, then rinse out. This shampoo will not only clean but also provide a wonderful herbal treatment each time you use it. Chamomile does have the power to lighten hair. If you would like to maintain your lovely dark tresses, use rosemary instead.

Lavender Shampoo

1/2 cup commercial, non-scented shampoo

1/3 cup spring water

4 tablespoons dried lavender or lavender tea

5 drops lavender essential oil (optional)

Bring the water to a boil and pour over the dried lavender. Allow it to steep for up to 15 minutes. Strain off the dregs and add the liquid to the soap and essential oil mixture. Place in a large glass container with a lid and shake well. It may need to be stirred or shaken before each use.

Natural Hair Color for Blondes

1/2 cup dried chamomile flowers

5 drops chamomile essential oil

Juice of 1½ lemons

1/2 teaspoon pure lemon extract (optional)

1/2 tablespoon lemon zest (peel)

4 cups spring water

Bring the water to a boil and pour over the combined ingredients. Stir and allow the mixture to steep for 15 minutes. Strain off the plant material and soak your hair in this concoction for at least 20 minutes. You may also pour the mixture over your hair repeatedly for 20 minutes. Rinse your hair well and allow it to air dry, preferably in the sun. Honey, beer or white wine vinegar may also be added to the colorant.

Natural Hair Color for Redheads

1/2 cup calendula (marigold) flowers

1 teaspoon carrot essential oil (optional)

1 tablespoon pure cherry extract (optional)

2 tablespoons red wine vinegar (optional)

2 cups spring water

Natural Hair Color for Redheads (continued)

Follow the directions as specified for "Natural Hair Color for Blondes."

Natural Hair Color for Brunettes

1/2 cup dried rosemary

1 teaspoon translucent henna powder (optional)

5 drops rosemary essential oil (optional)

3 bags black tea

1 cup prepared black coffee or espresso

Follow the directions as specified for "Natural Hair Color for Blondes." Blackstrap molasses may also be added for extra conditioning and highlights.

Natural Highlights for White Hair

3 tablespoons translucent henna powder

10 drops Roman blue chamomile essential oil

1 cup spring water

Follow the directions as specified for "Natural Hair Color for Blondes."

Petal Hair Treatment

1/2 cup fresh rose petals

5 drops rose essential oil

1/2 tablespoon rose water flavoring extract (optional)

1 egg, beaten

1/4 cup white rum

Heat the rum and add the rose petals. Allow the mixture to cool and steep overnight. The next day, remove the plant material and add the beaten egg, extract and essential oil. Beat well with a whisk. A 1/4 cup of water may also be added at this time. Apply to your hair, paying special attention to the ends. Leave on up to 30 minutes. Rinse off well with shampoo. Extra conditioning isn't required afterwards.

Aromatic Tresses

Having fragrant hair is not a new concept. For ages, women would use flowers or perfume to add a pleasant scent to their hair. By using commercial, perfumed shampoos that mimic designer fragrances or fresh flowers one can easily *wash* the scent in. But that is all it is many times: just scent. Why not use scent and healing combined with essential oils for a nice change? The great part about essential oils, especially the undiluted, Aromatherapy-grade kind, is they can very easily be added to commercial products. About 10 drops (less if you have sensitivities) is all you need. Having real rose shampoo or lavender conditioner can't get much easier. There are a number of essential oils specifically indicated for hair. They include:

- Geranium (be careful, it can lighten)
- Rosemary (be careful, this darkens hair)
- Lemon
- Lavender

Actually, almost all of the essential oils can be used on the hair; however, depending on your specific needs, some will work better. One also has to be careful of the lightening and darkening effects that some essential oils may have on your hair.

One essential oil I have found to do wonders is oregano. If you do not have the essential oil, you can use the fresh or dried sort from your cupboard. For many years Italian women have been using it on their hair to make it lustrous and it truly does do so. Like rosemary, however, it can slightly darken your hair. I used 5 drops in about 1 cup of filtered water and allowed it to sit 1 day before using it. You can also add a capful of vanilla extract for an absolutely glorious scent combination. It works best after washing your hair and substantially reduces tangles and frizzes in summer! It is quite amazing.

Another great oil for hair is lemon. It has the reverse effects of oregano, and sometimes lightens the hair if one spends much time outdoors in the sun. Not only does it make your hair smell very clean, it removes oil build-up, which is especially a problem in the summer time. Of course, if you would like some nice natural highlights, you can place the lemon oil in some spring water, toss in a bit of fresh zest as well, and place it in an atomizer or small spray bottle. After you wash your hair, spray where desired and let your hair air dry. Sitting in the sun isn't needed . . . it gives you a headache anyway. Walking outdoors without a hat on a sunny day while completing chores will suffice.

If you mix the lemon with other fruits and florals (grapefruit, orange, nerolie, jasmine, etc.), the effect can be out of this world. Please note, however, that bees may find your hair just as exciting. Tone down the florals in summer to help prevent attracting the wrong type of attention.

Chapter 9

AGELESS SECRETS
for
YOUNGER LOOKING SKIN

Bringing the Spa Home

All right, let me appeal to the vanity in us all. Let's face it, the image we project to the public reflects how we feel inside. Did you know that patients who come to the doctor's office with make up, freshly pressed clothes and their hair done are often made to wait longer? This is because you don't "appear" sick! Other more scruffy patients may easily be taken ahead of you due to the fact that you do not look as ill as the rest. Caring about how we look is more than just vanity, though. If you look at the mentally disturbed and depressed, they often have very little interest in their outward appearance. This is not normal because humans are social creatures. A whole industry has grown up around our desire to look and smell good, adding to our convivial appeal.

The Lipstick Test

Far from being a clinical assay, the Lipstick Test is a name given to female patients who are starting to "come around" after a bout of illness. While in the hospital, women who are very sick will often neglect their appearance. They just do not feel well enough to care for these extra personal things. However, as the patient begins to feel better, she may ask for a hand mirror and, yes, . . . some lipstick! This is an excellent sign of her progressive recovery.

The same philosophy applies to breast cancer survivors. Patients will many times lose their hair, healthy coloring and weight due to the chemotherapy. It is really a low point for many very sick women to witness vestiges of their femininity disappear. For a woman, hair loss alone is often devastating. The Nazi concentration camps shaved both men and women's heads for a reason. That reason was to make them feel vulnerable and weak. Therefore, losing our crowning glory is a reason for depression in and of itself.

That is why there are services and classes specifically designed to show women how to use wigs, make-up and prosthetic breast forms to make them look better. It is well known that when you look better, you will feel better. Depression due to any source causes the immune system to break down, which decreases your chances for healing. It is too soon to say, but it appears that increased survival rates for breast cancer patients may be correlated to women who took advantage of these optional programs during treatment and recovery.

Skin Care as We Age

This chapter will provide some wonderful formulas for clear, smooth, moist skin at any age. If you are already entering menopause, keep in mind that diminished estrogen production will automatically affect the look of your skin. Most often you may notice a thinning of the dermis, the layer of skin under the epidermis. What this means is that less estrogen will cause less oil and collagen to be produced. Therefore, the outer layer begins to sag and not "fit" snugly the way it used to. This is why getting a face-lift may not solve all of your problems. It is the structure under the skin that also needs reinforcing.

Unfortunately, much of the hype about products that include collagen and elastin are just that. The molecules of these substances are just too large to penetrate the epidermis. They may have moisturizing qualities, but they can not penetrate the skin to do very much good where it is needed. You will find yourself paying thousands of dollars at the make-up counter for products that do little more than sit on top of the skin. This is not to say that nothing works. There are a few products and non-surgical procedures out there that give excellent results for less than you would pay at the Chanel counter:

Glycolic Acid Peels

This is an in-office procedure that is less caustic than the stronger phenols. It utilizes concentrated fruit acids to slough off the top layer of skin and encourage new cellular growth from deep within. The result is smaller pores, smoother skin, diminished freckles and a luminous glow. This treatment will not remove deep wrinkles or creases, but fine lines virtually disappear. Dermatologists use a stronger percentage of the glycolic acid than salons can acquire. They also have more training to deal with reactions such as irritations and burns. While rare, these side effects can occur in sensitive patients. You do not want someone putting this kind of chemical on your face and then running off to check on another client's perm! Skip the salon, go to the dermatologist's office. One such plastic surgeon who offers this procedure at his Matawan, New Jersey office is Dr. Paul M. Goldberg. "These peels are effective in addressing fine lines and wrinkles. It is an excellent alternative to some of the more invasive procedures such as dermabrasion yet still offers smoothing and firming of the skin without the associated risks."

Generally the procedure begins with an office visit once a week for 10 weeks for the mini-peels. Once the skin has been conditioned, the only maintenance required is having the peels done once every six weeks or so. The results are often just short of miraculous. They include a luminous glow, even skin tone, reduction of fine lines and wrinkles, tighter, firmer skin and a farewell to acne breakouts all in the same package. Incredible.

Microdermabrasion

Cleopatra was perhaps one of the first women recorded to have done this as part of her skin care routine. Microdermabrasion involves scraping the outer layer of dead skin cells off so that more youthful cells can come to the surface. You see, as we age, new skin cells come to the surface at an increasingly slower rate. By the time they do surface, they are already aged! I know this does not sound comforting, but the fact is everything slows down as we get older. However, we can give our skin some assistance to keep it smooth and vibrant at any age.

Movie stars have gone to Beverly Hills spas to have microdermabrasion done for years. This involves a unit that acts like a sandblaster in that it shoots aluminum oxide crystals onto the surface of your skin. Like sandblasting, it easily removes the top layer of dead skin cells in a mechanical, rather than a chemical, method. The operator sprays a fine mist of Aluminum Oxide crystals onto your skin and the excess is vacuumed up. It is important that the operator wear a face mask to prevent inhaling the airborne dust. DermaMed makes a unit for such microdermabrasion procedures and I highly recommend it for several reasons. First of all, this unit uses closed container cartridges. As a closed system, this machine vacuums up the contaminated or used Aluminum oxide crystals and holds them in a sealed container. Other units may actually spray back used crystals from previous patients! This kind of cross-contamination should be avoided, of course.

The results are very similar to the glycolic acid peels mentioned previously, but there is no burning and you can see the results *after only one treatment*. Many doctor's offices are bringing in this equipment to serve their patients since microdermabrasion is very helpful for acne scarring as well as fine lines and wrinkles. There is also an excellent unit that can be used at home called the DermaNew™ Personal Microdermabrasion System. It uses the same Corundum crystals as do the $12,000.00 machines, but they are contained in a creme so there is no chance of aerosolization, or blowing into the air. Perhaps best of all is that the DermaNew™ System can be used to augment any skin care program. You are also in complete control of how long and how often you choose to employ microdermabrasion. It is much, much cheaper than glycolic acid peels since it can be done in the privacy of your own home.

I have personally used the DermaNew™ system and the results were breathtaking after only one use. My skin continues to improve and the fine lines around my mouth and eyes are completely gone after only a few weeks of use. Even better is the fact that my skin is tighter, smoother and firmer . . . absolutely luminous! I have taken good care of my skin so I do not have sun damage or freckles. If you have been naughty in your youth with too much sunbathing, it may take a bit longer to achieve similar results. However a more economical and efficacious way of renewing aging skin you will not find elsewhere.

Natural Spa Treatments . . . for Pennies!

There are a few natural at home facials that can be used based on the benefits of naturally occurring glycolic acid. These "fruit" acids are present in milk, sugar cane and many other edibles. Don't laugh. People spend top dollar to receive such treatments, which are all the rage at posh beauty spas across the country. Using fruits, essential oils and botanicals they offer a refreshing change of pace for both you and your skin.

So, since you have been so good, I am going to share some of their pricey secrets for beautiful skin from head to toe. The following formulas are reprinted from *Secret Potions, Elixirs and Concoctions: Botanical & Aromatic recipes for Mind, Body & Soul* written by my daughter (yes, I am that old), Marie A. Miczak. This book is available from your local bookseller or contact the publisher at www.lotuspress.com. Just don't blame me if you start speaking with a French accent, crave Perrier and demand winter trips to the Riviera.

Secret Potions, Elixirs & Concoctions: Skin & Body Care

A great number of posh spas are now using "natural" and "botanical based" treatments. Some are even prepared fresh on site. The problem comes with the fact that many people do not have the funds to pay the ridiculous fees charged by some establishments. If they are able to pay, they can only afford to be pampered once or twice a year, on special occasions perhaps. Some treatments need to be applied on a regular basis before you start to notice a real difference. Finally, many people do not have the inclination or the time to trudge into a spa for a whole day. To remedy this, many spas and cosmetic companies are now producing and marketing products to use at home. Unfortunately these products can be quite expensive as well and do not use 100% pure and natural ingredients.

The only real way to know exactly what you are putting on your skin is to make the product yourself. Of course you can not make everything at home, but little by little you will find yourself replacing store bought items with the sensuously pleasing ones found in this book.

And now . . . the Formulas:

Body Care

Honeysuckle Body Elixir

   1 cup fresh honeysuckle flowers

   2 cups spring or distilled water

   1 teaspoon pure vanilla extract

In a small pot bring the water to a boil, reduce heat to very low and add flowers. Turn the heat off completely after 10 minutes. Cover the mixture and let stand on the stove for 5 hours. When done strain off all of the plant material and place in a clean glass bottle. Use as an all over body mist or in clay masks. Keep all unused portions refrigerated for no longer than a week.

Variations:

Try these recipes for your specific skin needs.

Gentle:

   1 cup fresh or ½ cup dried rose petals

   1 cup water

Rose is extremely gentle for sensitive skin. Use after a bath for a real treat.

Refreshing:

   2 tablespoons lemon zest

   1 cup water

   1 teaspoon vanilla extract

This formula works great in the morning after a shower to help awaken your senses.

Moisturizing:

   1 cup fresh or ½ cup dried rose petals

   1 cup water

   1 teaspoon banana extract

   5 drops rose essential oil (optional)

Placing body elixirs in mist bottles will make it easier for you to use and enjoy them.

Amazon Rain

> 4 cups spring or distilled water
>
> 1/2 teaspoon honey
>
> 10 drops coconut fragrance oil or 2 teaspoons coconut extract
>
> 1/2 teaspoon pure vanilla extract
>
> 5 drops jasmine essential oil

Mix all of the ingredients together and place in a spray bottle. Shake it well before using. This is a wonderful, lightly scented mist that you can use as you exercise or after a day of outdoor fun. Keep all unused portions in the refrigerator for no longer than a week.

Cleopatra's Milk Bath

> 2 cups dry milk powder
>
> 1/2 cup cornstarch
>
> 5 drops sandalwood essential oil
>
> 1/2 teaspoon pure vanilla extract
>
> One square piece of cheesecloth

Mix all of the ingredients in a small bowl until well incorporated. Place half of the recipe in the middle of the cheesecloth square, forming a mound. Bring the four corners together and tie with a piece of string. Run a hot bath and place the bag under the running water. When the bath has cooled to a comfortable temperature, gently squeeze the bag. At the end of the bath, quickly shower off any milk residue.

Shanghai Salts

2 cups cornstarch

1 cup rice flour

1/2 teaspoon ground cinnamon

1/4 tablespoon ground dried ginger

1 tablespoon cloves

10 drops essential orange oil

1/2 cup Epsom salts

1 to 2 drops yellow food coloring

Place all ingredients in a blender and mix well. Put 4 tablespoons in hot running water. Spicy and exotic, this is sure to become one of your favorite treats. Small candy jars with lids make the perfect containers. Store in a cool, dry place.

Crystal Salts

1/2 cup sea salt

1 cup baking soda

1/2 cup Epsom salts

20 drops lemongrass essential oil

A few drops red food coloring (optional)

Mix all of the ingredients together until completely blended. Place the mixture in a pretty glass bottle using a natural seashell from the shore as a measuring scoop. Store in a cool, dry place.

Love Bath

1 cup freshly picked rose petals

1/2 cup dried milk

10 drops rose essential oil

1 cheesecloth square

Combine all of the ingredients in a bowl. Transfer the

mixture to the cheesecloth, forming a mound in the center. Bring the four corners together and tie them with a piece of string. Run the bath water steaming hot and place the bag under the running water. When the bath is at a comfortable temperature, squeeze the bag a couple of times before entering.

Peppermint Candy Soak

    2 cups spring or distilled water
    1/2 cup loose peppermint tea or 2 tea bags
    1/2 cup Epsom salts
    10 drops peppermint essential oil

Bring the water to a boil and add the tea. Turn the heat off and steep for 1 or 2 hours, depending on the strength you desire. Remove the tea bags and place all of the ingredients in a blender until well incorporated. Clean glass bottles with corks or tops work best as containers. When ready to use, give the bottle a good shake and pour as much as you wish into the bath water. Store all unused portions in your refrigerator for no more than 2 weeks. It is great for sore, tired feet as well. It is very invigorating, so do not use it at night unless you are going dancing!

Mermaid's Lagoon

    1 cup Epsom salts
    1 cup coarse sea salt
    10 drops frangipani fragrance or essential oil
    10 drops blue food coloring

Combine all of the ingredients well and place in a container with a lid. Epsom salts do have the tendency to evaporate. Light and refreshing, this will quickly become one of your favorite indulgences.

Star Burst

1 cup Epsom salts

1 cup baking soda

20 drops strawberry fragrance oil

10 drops yellow food coloring

1 vanilla bean, split open

Mix the first four ingredients together in a large bowl. The reason this recipe calls for yellow food coloring instead of red is because these salts are supposed to smell like delicious star fruit. Unfortunately, star fruit scents aren't easily accessible so strawberry will suffice. Place the mixture in a clean container, pushing the vanilla bean straight down the center. With time the vanilla bean will add a warm touch to your Star Burst salts. Let cure 2 weeks before using. Store in a cool, dry place in a container with a tight fitting lid.

Queen of the Night Body Butter

8 tablespoons jojoba or sweet almond oil (base)

1 teaspoon vitamin E

1 tablespoon margarine

10 drops jasmine essential oil

3 drops vanilla essential oil

1/2 teaspoon honey

1 teaspoon natural bees wax

Place all of the ingredients in a saucepan. Mix until completely combined and melted. Turn the heat off and pour the mixture into a clean jar. Cover and place in the refrigerator. You may need to blend it a bit before using. A little goes a long way.

Complete Body Treatments

With this set of treatments you can turn your home into a lavish spa for a day. Be sure to review all of the steps prior to proceeding. Make adjustments to the concoctions depending on your skin type.

Almond Body Polisher

    4 tablespoons baking soda

    1/2 cup white corn meal

    10 natural almonds

    1 tablespoon almond extract

Place the almonds in a coffee grinder and pulse until ground well. The same can be achieved in a blender. Blend all of the ingredients together and store in the refrigerator until ready to use.

Rose Water Clay Mask

    1 cup rose Body Elixir

    5 drops rose essential oil (optional)

    Enough dry clay to make a thick mask

    1 teaspoon sweet almond or olive oil

Stir the ingredients together well and store in a clean container. Place the mixture in the refrigerator until ready to use.

Cherry Bath Oil

    4 tablespoons olive oil

    2 tablespoons canola oil

    2 tablespoons sweet almond oil

    1/2 teaspoon vitamin E

    10 drops cherry fragrance oil

In a small bowl mix all of the ingredients together. Keep refrigerated until ready to use.

Violet Body Splash

  2 cups fresh violet flowers
  3 cups spring or distilled water
  1/2 teaspoon vanilla extract

Heat the water to a boil. Add the flower petals and simmer for 15 minutes, covered. Turn the heat off and let sit for 1 hour. Pour the mixture into a glass container or ceramic cup and keep it refrigerated until ready to use. Strain off plant material and add the vanilla extract. If fresh violets are not in season, use one of the other Body Elixirs.

Step one:
Wet your skin before applying the Almond Body Scrub. Apply the scrub and gently massage in a circular motion to remove any dead skin. Rinse the scrub off with warm water.

Step two:
Apply the Rose Water Clay Mask to your arms, legs, thighs, etc. Be sure to avoid sensitive skin areas. Spread on a thin layer and let it dry for about 20 minutes.

Step three:
Draw a warm bath and add the Cherry Bath Oil. When the water is a comfortable temperature enter and soak until the clay can be wiped off easily with a wash cloth.

Step four:
Douse yourself quickly with the Violet Body Splash. If you like you can use the Queen of the Night Body Butter for an additional moisturizing effect.

Note: Always remember to do a patch test.

Facial Formulas

Youth in a Bottle

  10 drops rose essential oil

  10 drops neroli essential oil

  10 drops orange essential oil

  1 cup spring water

Place the ingredients in a bottle in the order listed, taking care to use a very clean glass bottle. Shake well before applying to freshly washed skin. Please do not substitute any of the essential oils for fragrance oils. The affect of this treatment will not be the same.

Rose Oil Rejuvenator

  10 drops rose essential oil

  2 tablespoons sweet almond oil

  3 drops geranium essential oil

Mix the ingredients well. Store the mixture in a glass bottle in the refrigerator. Use as a spot treatment for wrinkles and/or fine lines or as an all over face moisturizer. Do not use around the eyes.

Rose Facial Steam

  1/2 cup fresh or ¼ cup dried rose petals

  5 drops rose essential oil (optional)

  1/2 teaspoon vanilla extract

  Enough water to fill a large bowl

Using a tea kettle bring the water to a rolling boil. Place a large bowl on a hard, flat surface such as a table. Add the petals, extract and essential oil. Drape a bath towel over your head and pour the water into the bowl. Move your face as close as possible to the steam without burning yourself. If the steam is too hot, allow it to cool a bit.

Remain under the towel for about 20 to 30 minutes. Use no more than once a week.

European Milk Cleanser

2 cups dried milk

1 vanilla bean (optional)

5 drops lavender

Mix the ingredients together and place in a container with a lid. Store in a cool, dark place. To use the cleanser, moisten a small amount in your hand with water and smooth over your face and neck. Use the balls of your fingers to make small circular motions over your skin. Rinse well with warm water. Not only will this cleanse your skin but it will also help even-out your complexion.

Strawberry Yogurt Mask

1/4 cup plain yogurt

3 fresh strawberries

3 drops lavender essential oil

Remove the green leaves and stems from the strawberries. Using a fork smash them into a fine pulp. You can also use a blender or a small food processor. Mix in the yogurt and essential oil. Smooth the mixture over clean skin and leave it on for 15 to 20 minutes. Wash off with warm water. You will find this mask to be quite soothing and cooling to the skin. Discard any unused portions.

Chapter 10

CARING FOR OURSELVES AS WE GROW OLDER

Older Americans are the fastest growing segment of the American population. According to the Data Base *News in Aging* from the U.S. Census Bureau, we have seen a steep increase in the population of people aged 65 and older with a projection of 34.7% of the population by the end of the year 2000. People are living longer and what's better is that we are experiencing a higher quality of life. Surviving into our golden years is quickly being replaced with thriving. Still, seniors face the added challenges in physical and mental health, obtaining proper nutrition and retaining social independence.

Many older Americans continue to work past retirement, sometimes due to economic necessity, but often because their employment gives them purpose in life. Volunteer work is also on the rise with many senior citizens stepping forward to fill the void that social services often leave as a result of funding restraints. Still, respect for the value of this segment of the population is wanting. It can be seen no more blatantly than in the current health care system.

Consider this. Every hospital in the United States has a Pharmacy and Therapeutics Committee comprised of doctors, pharmacists and administrators. This committee decides what medications a hospital or nursing home will use on a regular basis, thus limiting the variety of drugs that specific facility has available. The medications selected by this council are called formulary drugs and doctors are encouraged to prescribe them ahead of more costly or even superior therapies. This all saves the facility money, but do you think it will be easy for a doctor to recommend an unapproved non-formulary drug specifically for an elderly patient? Even if a doctor orders a non-formulary drug in the best interest of the patient, he or she may need to get permission to use it. Considering that many of the Pharmacy and Therapeutics Committee members are non-medical hospital administrators, the emphasis can shift from what is best for the patient to what is best for the hospital's bottom line. Doctors and pharmacists on the committee may voice strong concerns, but they may still be categorized as hospital personnel in the eyes of the board. The hospital administrators, who often have no background in medicine, are considered the watchdogs for the hospital's viability as a business. As with any business, holding down costs and seeking out generous benefactors is imperative. Their job is not to cure but to keep the hospital afloat by conserving resources. Their professional rewards come from doing this efficiently and keeping the institution in the black.

This obviously spills over into decisions that effect patient care. For example, look at a prescription. It is a legal document. If you look at the lower portion of the script, you will see a box that reads, "Do Not Substitute" and "Substitution Permissible." This judgment call is the physician's prerogative based upon what he knows about the drug's available proprietary and generic forms and what would be best for the patient. Cost factors may be a reason to allow for a generic substitution in consideration of the financial status of his patient. Still, the physician who is knowledgeable of their patient's need should make these decisions, not an HMO or managed care.

Often times deals are made with drug wholesalers and generic drug manufacturers to cut costs. Increasingly, many HMO's have *their* own pharmacy that limits the doctor's choices even more. Many generic drug manufacturers have products that differ in bioequivalence to their proprietary counterparts, or even another generic product from a more reputable company. There are documented cases of vast differences in bioequivalency between the same generic drug manufactured by different companies. Since problems of equal effectiveness are often reported in peer reviewed pharmaceutical journals, the general public seldom sees these findings. To see how these variations can affect patient outcomes, consider the following scenario:

You have been taking Synthroid® for many years. Your thyroid is now dysfunctional and produces little or none of its own thyroxine. Your HMO changes you over to the generic form of the drug, which is called levothyroxine sodium. A cheap generic drug manufacturer supplies it. This company uses inexpensive binders, fillers, excipients and glazing agents that inhibit optimal absorption of the medication in the small intestines. Even though you are taking your standard milligram dosage, you notice sluggishness, intolerance to cold, weight gain, etc. You complain to your doctor about these newly emerging symptoms, but because you are over 60, your doctor tells you not to worry since such things can be expected as you get older. Subsequently you are putting on even more weight and what is left of your fine gray hair is becoming brittle, dry and falling out. Once again you voice your concerns to your physician but he mildly counters that you are getting older and these things are common to geriatric patients. Since he is so convinced that your symptoms are solely due to the aging process (or even your imagination,) he never orders the customary thyroid panel that would routinely be considered for a younger person.

Even though generic drugs must demonstrate bioavailability and bioequivalence through clinical assays and testing submitted to the FDA, there has been a notable compromise between generics manufactured by different companies according to *U.S. Pharmacist*, a peer reviewed pharmacy journal.

Society's perception of the elderly accounts for most of this. Yet, you cannot just stand there and take it. You must speak up for yourself if you are to expect and receive quality health care. Just look at the apathetic attitude towards health exhibited by many nursing homes, even the private ones. As far as nutrition, how many elderly nursing home residents who are diagnosed as borderline diabetics receive white bread, Jell-O®, juice, peanut butter and jelly, yogurt and Ensure® . . . all in the same meal? It is far more common than you think. The registered dietitian's retort? "Well, that's all he'll eat." So food quantity weighs far above food quality and nourishment is replaced with simply feeding.

All calculated, this meal is practically all sucrose or simple sugar with few nutrients to show for the caloric intake. However, like the hospital formulary of approved drugs, these foods win out in part because they fit the budgetary requirement of the nursing home. Adding insult to injury, all of this refined sugar stresses the insulin production from the pancreas. Type II Diabetics often advance to requiring insulin as a result. Once again, you have the right and duty to yourself to ask that all meal plans be reviewed for health and nutritional value. Otherwise, in place of preventative medicine, you will have the dull acceptance of the mediocre without optimal health in your advancing years.

There is factual evidence that adequate nutrition is indeed quite difficult for many elderly patients to obtain due to biochemical changes effecting digestion. For example, have you noticed that perhaps when you were young you could drink quarts of milk with no problem? Perhaps when you got older, you cut back on milk and other dairy products due to the fat content. Now if you drink a glass of milk it makes you gassy and may even upset your stomach. This is because when you were younger, one of the enzymes your digestive system produced in abundance was lactase. Lactase works primarily on the substrate lactose, or milk sugar, which is present in dairy products.

Our bodies are very stingy about enzyme production. If you do not consume products with lactose, your body will not burden itself with the production of lactase to break it down. Products such as Lactaid® work because the lactase is built into the product. This just begins to scratch the surface of diminished enzyme production and its correlation with the aging process. All you need do is look at a child. They can eat all sorts of wild combinations of foods at one time. You will seldom hear them belch or complain of gas or bloating. This is because youngsters produce adequate quantities of digestive enzymes that allow them to make quick work of breaking down their food and absorbing most of the nutrients present. As we get older, that which is not digested ferments, and you know the consequences of that process . . . flatulence!

There is another component to digestion and absorption of nutrients. According to health officials, of particular concern to seniors should be the B complex vitamins. An estimated 30% of seniors lose their ability to make stomach acid and this interferes with the absorption of vitamin B-12 and folic acid. Studies suggest that deficiencies in these as well as in vitamin B-6 can cause neurological changes such as a decline in alertness, loss of memory and numbness in the extremities. B-2, or riboflavin, aids in the release of energy from carbohydrates, proteins and fats. Adding to this is the fact that many elderly people take medications regularly. Some of these medications can lead to deficiencies, especially if taken continuously.

Ultimately there is a change in absorption of nutrients as we age due to the decrease in digestive enzyme production. Even though older patients may be consuming a variety of foods, the utilization of nutrients contained therein may still be compromised. While this is no medical mystery, many health professionals still scratch their heads in disbelief when they see affluent senior citizens in a state of malnutrition. Refusing to acknowledge these special needs and differences among the aged, the same non-workable solutions are set forth with unsuccessful results in improving nutritional status and health.

Those who can go elsewhere for a second opinion usually do. As for those institutionalized in nursing homes and hospitals, registered dietitians are usually hired to oversee the planning of meals. It is interesting to observe that when malnutrition is seen in these settings, the patient is often blamed for not eating the unpalatable fare of canned and refined foods. High sucrose feeding formulas are then quickly instituted. Now the companies are even getting you used to the inevitable by marketing these liquid-feeding formulas to people who are healthy and non-institutionalized! Each person will have to decide based on the subjective facts, "Is this the best nutritional program for me?" Do not allow age to be a factor in your decision. Whether you are 5 or 95 you need and deserve fresh, enzyme-rich, whole foods to thrive. We should not accept the common misconception that we should expect less as we get older because that is exactly what we will receive.

There is also the challenge of preserving mental health, which is also closely associated with diet and nutrition. High blood pressure can lead to memory loss and diminished cognitive ability, which are often seen in the elderly.

Another area of mental health to be concerned about is the onset of late life depression. Where the person lives and his or her level of independence is often a major factor. For example, elderly people who are regular community residents have a prevalence of late life depression between 3-5%. These are the people you see in your neighborhood going about their own business, maybe a little more slowly than the rest but still living independently. In stark contrast, studies conducted in nursing homes show major depression affecting 15-25% of residents in that setting. This means that up to one in every four nursing home residents is diagnosed with clinical depression. What is worse is many elderly patients initially diagnosed with minor depression will go on to develop major depression while institutionalized. This study comes on the heels of growing issues concerning the use of antidepressants in long-term care facilities and the geriatric patient.

The combined factors of poor nutrition, decreased absorption, multiple medication regimes and mental depression pose very specific health concerns for the elderly. According to the *New York Times* over 100,000 people die of drug interactions every year in the U.S. Since the potential for interactions between medicines, herbs and vitamins are not well known, how many more have died without proper diagnosis? The Food and Drug Administration collects reports on adverse drug and supplement interactions, but has to hope that doctors and pharmacists will report such cases. As a result, only about 1 percent of such incidents are even reported to the FDA. The others simply fall by the wayside because the actual cause of the bad interaction may be uncertain. Many times if the patient is elderly, once again, it is presumed they died of natural causes when perhaps the underlying reason was a drug interaction.

To provide an example, a man with a replacement heart valve almost developed a lethal blood clot when he began taking ginseng (*Panax, ginseng*). To prevent blood from collecting around his newly implanted heart valve, he was taking warfarin sodium, a blood thinner also known as Coumadin®. He took the herbal ginseng supplements three times daily for two weeks. During a routine follow up visit, his physician's test revealed dangerously thick blood. He stopped taking the ginseng and after two weeks his blood's clotting level returned to normal. Thus the correlation was drawn that perhaps the ginseng inactivated the blood-thinning medication.

How many times have you heard someone say "Yeah, the doctors aren't quite sure what he died of, but you know, he was pretty old anyway." So we shouldn't even bother to investigate? Of course we should, but this is an example of how pervasive this kind of thinking is to the point that we accept the rationale without question. We should not accept that sickness, depression and poor health are a "natural" part of the aging process. Scientific research has told us that often times most diseases are not attributable to age. One great example is Alzheimer's disease. This was often categorized incorrectly as senile dementia and accepted as a part of getting old. However, even though the onset and frequency of the disease does increase with age, younger people have been diagnosed with this disease as well. This is one way that medical researchers discovered that Alzheimer's was not a normal part of the aging process, but an abnormal attack and destruction of brain cells. As a result, more effort is being put into the study and treatment of this disease. An abnormality may be easier to conquer than an inevitable part of aging.

We can't be sure how many other conditions commonly attributed to aging may actually be abnormalities caused by disease or other factors. Until then we should approach health problems in the elderly the same way as we do the young, with optimism. We must first identify and work on the treatable conditions to see if this brings any improvement. Next, look at what can be improved in the patient's diet and exercise regimen. Facilitators at assisted living communities have noted that patients given proper nutrition may actually "come back" from what was seen as a downward decline in mental function and memory retention. All people need interaction. Just the act of participating in normal conversation is very validating to our sense of self-respect and worth in society. People of all ages need to know that their opinions count for something and what they think still matters.

While there is no cure for Alzheimer's yet and its etiology is not clearly understood there are many things that you can do to sharpen your mental acuity no matter what your current status. Engaging in events and activities that stimulate the mind are at the top of the list of lifestyle adjustments. Sitting alone with the television on day and night is a sure way to lose your edge. Instead, try crossword puzzles. They make you think in very abstract terms and can keep the gray matter in the pink. Also, hobbies can be very useful. Painting, sculpting, sewing and knitting all require creative, abstract thought processes. This allows an individual to step outside the realm of the mundane day to day cycle and be inventive. Not only does this impact a person's sense of accomplishment, there is an increase in self esteem. Many elders begin to feel "old and worthless" if they are not allowed to contribute something. Families need to encourage participation, allowing older members to do what they can to help within their abilities. If something isn't done just right, do not make an issue of possibly having to do the job over. It is the effort that counts.

If you are experiencing mild problems with short-term memory, one formula taken from *Nature's Weeds, Native Medicine* can help in increasing blood flow to the brain, which often diminishes in our 60s. It can be given as a hot infusion or tea or ground up and placed into gelatin capsules. Hard-pressed herbal tablets are generally not recommended, especially for the elderly. This is because older people often lack the hydrochloric stomach acid to break them down. Hence many of these pills end up being passed out of the body unabsorbed.

Natural Brain Power Blend

> 1/2 cup dried basil
> 1/8 cup dried rosemary
> 1/4 cup dried peppermint leaves

Grind the dried leaves together until fine. Place in a teaball and steep in one pint of freshly boiled water for 3-5 minutes.

The peppermint stimulates the brain while the basil and rosemary heighten mental function and mental alertness. Rosemary is also a fantastic antioxidant, protecting the brain cells from the ravages of naturally occurring free radicals. It is a wonderful aid for memory retention. Just don't use it at night, it'll keep you wide awake! To this protocol, you might add a standardized ginkgo biloba concentrate. This may be taken with or without the tea. However, once again, stay away from the herbal tablets of ginkgo. They are often too hard to break down for absorption. Try purchasing ginkgo in two piece gelatin capsules or even sealed soft gels. The will break down much more readily for assimilation in the small intestine and you will actually get your money's worth. A standardized product means that a certain percentage of the bioactive components of that herb are guaranteed in each bottle you buy. Some herbalists believe that this is not very important and that using the whole herb is. There may be something to this. Herbs are so very complex that we cannot really choose only one chemical component from the plant and say "this is the part that works." We can, however, make an educated guess and make sure the product has these bioactive components in addition to the whole herb. You will have the best of both worlds and a more complete herbal product.

You need to remember that when using herbs, potencies can vary from year to year according to soil and growing conditions, rainfall levels, and storage before processing. Some of the best herbal products come from plants that you have grown fresh yourself. After all, they are only "weeds" and highly competitive in reproducing in the wild. So you should find them quite easy to cultivate in a sunny window or patio box for your own use.

Suggested Supplementation for Older Women

Minerals:

1,200 - 1,500 mg calcium

200 mg magnesium

50 mcg selenium, a trace mineral

Digestive Enzymes:

Chewable papaya with enzymes, papain, lipase, protease, etc.

Vitamins:

Balanced B-complex supplement

500 mg esterized vitamin C

400 I.U. vitamin E (May temporarily increase blood pressure when first used.)

Daily multivitamin without iron

Herbs:

Standardized ginkgo biloba (Do not use if you are taking Coumadin®)

Wolfberry extract (*Lycium barbarum* fruit)

Standardized hawthorn berry concentrate (Use only under your health practitioner's care)

145

Avoid iron supplements or multivitamins with iron unless recommended by your doctor!

Ginkgo Biloba for a Lot More Than Just Memory!

Ginkgo biloba has captured the public's attention as the remedy for poor memory and mental acuity. Young executives state that ginkgo has provided them with a mental edge for better performance on the job. The truth is that for most people under the age of 65, ginkgo offers diminished returns in regard to increasing blood flow to the brain. This is because under age 65, most adults' blood flow is quite sufficient. You will not see a noticeable drop until after age 70 in most people! However, younger adults can still benefit from the antioxidant qualities of ginkgo. The ginkgo tree, or maidenhair tree, is very popular in urban areas because of its tolerance to smog and air pollution. The same antioxidant qualities that allow it to survive in such toxic environments make it quite appropriate for the same application in humans.

Still, ginkgo does a lot more than increase blood flow to the head and provide antioxidant protection against free radicals. A study published in the *Journal of Urology* showed ginkgo helps relieve impotence caused by narrowing of the arteries that supply blood to the penis. Sixty men with erection problems caused by impeded penile blood flow were given 60 milligrams of ginkgo a day. By the end of the year-long study half of the men regained erections. According to pharmacologist and author Varro Tyler ". . . there is an impressive body of literature attesting to the effectiveness of Ginkgo Biloba Extract (GBE) in treating ailments associated with decreased cerebral blood flow, particularly in geriatric patients. These conditions include short-term memory loss, headache, tinnitus, depression and the like. Both clinical and pharmacological studies have shown that Ginkgo Biloba Extract promotes vasodilation and improved blood flow in both the arteries and capillaries. There are also indications that it is an effective free radical scavenger. Large doses are required, which explains why a concentrate is used rather than the herb itself." Tyler goes on to state that the commonly used form is a concentrated extract, standardized to 24% flavonoids and 6% terpenes.

Herbalist Michael Hoffman cites research that shows ginkgo benefiting the normalization of blood pressure in the circulatory system. It appears that ginkgo reduces the tendency of clot formation in veins and arteries, suggesting use in the prevention of coronary thrombosis and in recovery from strokes and heart attacks. It has been shown to lower blood pressure and dilate peripheral blood vessels in patients recovering from thrombosis of blood clots. If you are currently on Coumadin® therapy you may soon see Ginkgo Biloba Extract (GBE) take center stage for both thrombosis prevention and blood pressure normalization.

Wolfberry – Potent Antioxidant

Coming from the Orient, we have wolfberry or as it is known by its Latin name, *Lycium barbarum*. Wolfberry is a member of the solanaceae family and grows as a wild bush in northwest China. Used as both fruit and medicine, wolfberry provides 19 amino acids, trace minerals and vitamin C specifically. It is touted to be one of the richest antioxidants available, neutralizing free radical peroxidation. The dried fruits are very pleasant tasting, therefore compliance will not be a problem. Preliminary studies have shown wolfberry to improve normal cell proliferation and restore and repair DNA, thus indicating it may prevent cancer. In fact, Japanese researchers reported wolfberry fruits could inhibit the growth of cancer cells. Wolfberry's dried fruits, as well as a concentrated extract, are available from Rich Nature™. You can visit their website at www.richnature.com or call 1-888-708-8127.

Hawthorn Berry for High Blood Pressure & Heart Disease

Another factor that is accepted as a part of getting older is the onset of high blood pressure. Practically every medical book will tell you that as we get older, the arteries begin to become coated and the lumen or inner diameter grows smaller. This constricted passageway does not allow the artery the normal flexing ability, therefore blood pressure will increase. Many blood pressure charts allow for this by citing normal blood pressure for a person aged 70 can be as high as 166/91. The focus is not correct. Why don't we question how the arteries became occluded in the first place and when this happens, what can be done to regain normal function to them? Scientific research into diets high in saturated fat or animal fat indicate that food choices most decidedly are the cause. In any event, no matter what has happened in the past, you have the opportunity to turn things around . . . today. An herb that is proving to be a valuable ally in the fight against heart disease and hypertension is hawthorn berry.

Hawthorn, *Crataegus* species of the rosaceae family, has been used for many years to treat heart failure in Europe. Active ingredients are extracted from the berries, leaves and flowers and include antioxidants such as quercetin and rutin.

Studies done in Czechoslovakia, the United States and Germany suggest hawthorn may benefit heart health on many levels. In lowering blood pressure, hawthorn acts by dilating the peripheral blood vessels, moderating heart rate and by mild ACE (angiotensin converting enzyme) inhibition. All of these add up to less stress on the heart and coronary arteries. Patients of the New York Heart Association's functional class II, which includes mild to moderate heart failure, were given a daily dose of 600 mg of hawthorn extract. After an eight-week period, study patients showed marked clinical improvement.

Caution should be taken, however, when using hawthorn along with digitalis-based heart medications such as Lanoxin (digoxin). This interaction may require a lowered dose of up to one half of the prescription drug. Hawthorn's benefits to the heart and blood pressure develop slowly, so it should not be used to treat acute angina attacks. Even so, studies have noted over time its potential usefulness in treating stable angina pectoris. People should be warned about self-medicating with hawthorn, especially for long periods of time since adverse reactions include hypotension or dangerously low blood pressure, fatigue, nausea and sedation with high doses. People who are allergic to the rosaceae family of plants or who are pregnant should not take hawthorn at all.

Chapter 11

THE MIND, BODY, SPIRIT CONNECTION

Self-Expression in the Textile Arts:
Spinning & Weaving – Natural Stress Relief
for Women!

Women all over the world face incredible stress everyday. In many industrialized nations, we are both the breadwinner and nurturer with all the many hats worn in between. Our place in developing countries often sees us rising with the sun and continuing long after dark with our chores. This is especially so in many agrarian, or agricultural-based, societies.

When I first began to write books on natural health and healing, I did so from a woman's perspective as far as needs and considerations. This is because our lifestyles often tie us so very closely to the heartbeat of the family. We often put our needs far behind those of our children and husbands, which results in great suffering. It is very difficult for us to sit down and forget about everything for an evening. Our chores, children and unfinished work call to us constantly and we respond.

However there are workable solutions. Right now I am working on a book dealing with holistic health options for women. I began to explore ways that women could engage in creative yet productive activities that would free them from the burden of day to day stress. Hence I was introduced to the textile arts, specifically spinning and weaving.

Female spinners and weavers that I interviewed have told me how relaxing and gratifying this activity is! Many likened spinning to a calming mantra. They spoke of how the rhythm of the wheel melds with the rotation of the universe. In weaving, there is a creation of artistically inspired fabrics only limited by one's imagination. The bonding factor between these two activities and women is that practically every culture has a method for spinning and weaving. The Incas of ancient Peru used a drop spindle to spin llama and alpaca fleece into fine garments befitting even their kings. Likewise many African tribes and nomadic nations will follow their herds, utilizing a wide variety of fleeces from their livestock.

Are you a material girl? Although I am but a novice spinner, I enjoyed the connection between women and generations when my daughter and I had our first lesson. I knew that my ancestors from England and Ireland had learned the same way. My Native American ancestors were woodland weavers, using the inner barks of trees that were softened, twisted and woven into bags, moccasins and many other useful items. Over and above being a peaceful pasttime, spinning and weaving have helped many women to become financially independent. As people have less and less time to make handmade items, the value of those items made by human hands is increasing. You need only go to a few upscale department stores to see the price of items that have tags indicating they were hand-made.

In recognizing this, perhaps women will look into the textile arts of spinning and weaving and find a happy medium. That would be the perfect balance of relaxation with creation. A woman can sit and spin, giving her mind a chance to focus on something other than the day to day grind of endless problems. When she is done, she has for her effort created a product, a skein of yarn that now can be utilized further to create whatever her imagination can allow. She then can take that yarn and crochet or weave an item that she personally wants or needs. A hat, blanket or a sweater . . . she is in total control of the fate of that skein of yarn. In that simple act, she is empowered because her creativity has a viable outlet and her imagination has a physical embodiment. Ultimately, her dreams have a tangible manifestation.

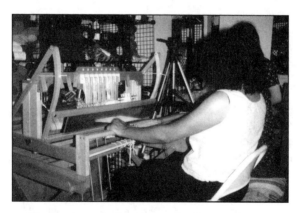

Weaving is not only a form of self-expression, but empowers women to create their own clothing.

I believe what Elizabeth Ashford is doing for the global community of women could well be emulated by many others. There is a saying "Give a man (or woman) a fish and he eats for a day. Teach a man to fish and he can feed himself and his family for the rest of his life." I would like to encourage everyone to continue supporting expansive programs like these for women. Spinning and weaving are so much more than idle pastimes. They have been the core of many women's existence, both emotionally and

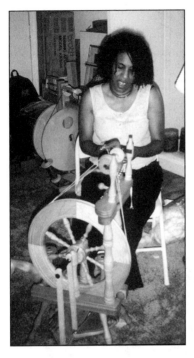

physically, for centuries. I think that in the years to come these activities will give us grounding in a world that is so volatile to change. That is the one link between our environment and what we are able to contribute and make of it.

Tulasi Kilgore
using the Ashford Traveller wheel.

For more information on getting started in the textile arts, visit The Joy of Handspinning, the Web Site for Handspinners at www.joyofhandspinning.com or e-mail Tulasi Kilgore at: info@joyofhandspinning.com. Tulasi is the owner of The Joy of Handspinning and a wonderful spinning and weaving teacher. Her website is a great place to begin to learn how to spin because it contains free video clips of techniques in the yarn making process. Tulasi also has a CD-ROM that walks you through the steps of setting up your wheel, of which there are several styles.

RESOURCES
& REFERENCES

API® Protective Ankle Inserts
1-902-854-3319
www.apihockey.com

Protective inserts for skating and skiing.

Belk & Associates, Inc.
1-803-957-6323
www.belkwigs.com

Hair loss solutions and the world's finest human hair wigs.

Cashmere Socks.com
1-212-724-6331
www.CashmereSocks.com

Buttery soft cashmere socks for sensitive feet and medical conditions of the extremities.

Clear Clouds™ by Skating Safe, Inc.

1-888-299-2553 (phone & fax)

www.SkatingSafe.com or e-mail Info@SkatingSafe.com

Gel ankle sleeves, disks and hip protectors for skating, skiing and other athletics.

FABS® for Foot Comfort

1-800-486-0325

www.DrRoths.com

Doctor-developed innovative strap-on arch supports that relieve heel pain, tired, achy feet and general leg and back pain.

GeorGie Wigs

1-888-GEORGIE

www.georgiewigs.com

The absolute finest human hair wigs in the world.

Graf Canada

1-888-703-GRAF (4723)

www.grafcanada.com

World class yet comfortable figure and hockey skates. Worn by Olympic champions such as Michelle Kwan.

Harmony Sports (PIC® Skates)

1-800-882-3448

www.picskate.com

The best inline, artistic skates made.

Klingbeil Shoe Labs Inc.

1-718-297-6864

www.klingbeilskatingboots.com

Beautiful, handmade stock and custom boots crafted for the individual skater's foot.

Light Force Therapy
1-888-259-9996
www.lightforcetherapy.com

Accu-Beam is cleared by the FDA to relieve pain from arthritis and help improve circulation.

Lotus Press
P.O. Box 325
Twin Lakes, WI 53181, USA
1-262-889-8561 (phone)
1-262-889-2461 (fax)
E-mail: lotuspress@lotuspress.com
Website: www.lotuspress.com

Publisher of books on Ayurveda, Reiki, aromatherapy, energetic healing, herbalism, alternative health and US editions of Sri Aurobindo's writings.

Dr. Marie Miczak
P.O. Box 312
Manalapan, NJ 07726
1-877-707-1970
www.miczak.com

Natural health & nutrition books, articles plus Dr. Miczak's Skin Care Renewal system featuring her Microdermabrasion Skin Care line of products.

Marie Anakee Miczak
www.anakee.com

Books on natural health and living, herbs and more – along with articles, art gallery and store.

Rich Nature™
1-888-708-8127

www.richnature.com

The most antioxidant fruit on earth. Dried Wolfberry concentrate and Wolfberry soap.

Riedell Skates
1-800-698-6893

www.riedellskates.com

Comfortable, heat-moldable boots for every level skater and traditional Mitchell King, John Wilson blades.

Rollerblade®
1-800-232-ROLL

www.rollerblade.com

The original women's specific fit, in-line skates for beginners to advanced skaters.

The Joy of Handspinning
www.joyofhandspinning.com or e-mail Tulasi Kilgore at: info@joyofhandspinning.com

Everything you need for spinning and weaving.

Tempur-Pedic® Mattress Co.
1-888-664-2036

www.tempurpedic.com

Pressure-relieving Swedish mattress and pillow.

Thorlos® for Every Activity
www.thorlo.com

Specialty athletic socks for practically every sports activity.

ABOUT THE AUTHOR

Marie Miczak, D.Sc., Ph.D. is an alumnus of Rutgers University College of Pharmacy. Dr. Miczak holds a doctorate in Nutrition Science and is certified with the American Association of Nutritional Consultants. She also holds a doctorate in a branch of Pharmacognosy (the study of medicines derived from plants and natural sources), and is a member of the American College of Clinical Pharmacology and the American Pharmaceutical Association's Academy of Science and Research.

Dr. Miczak is adjunct professor for Brookdale and Clayton Colleges as well as a visiting professor for universities across the nation. She is a frequent guest on network television, appearing as an expert in her chosen field of nutraceuticals on both TV and radio. Her syndicated columns are published and read internationally and she is the prolific author of over 4 books including *Nature's Weeds, Native Medicine* and *The Secret of Staying Young: Age Reversal for Mind & Body*, which are published by Lotus Press.

Dr. Miczak has written a series of books dedicated to protecting your health with little-known facts about adverse interactions and alternative medicine detailing both the benefits and the risks. The name of the series is *"How Not to Kill Yourself"* and is published by Random House.

The first title in this series is *How Not to Kill Yourself with Deadly Interactions . . . When Herbs, Drugs, Foods and Vitamins Don't Mix.* For more information about Dr. Miczak's courses or information regarding how to order her books visit her website: www.miczak.com.

To schedule a speaking engagement, interview or media appearance call toll free, 1-877-707-1970.

INDEX

Candida Albicans 12
chamomile 35, 71, 114
charlie horse 99
chasteberry 13
cherry 130
childbearing 31
chitin 68
chitosan 68
chromium picolinate 68
clover 13
cloves 127
clitoris 52
coconut 126
colds 38
conception 39

D

diabetes 71
dandelion 13
dream cycle 73

E

echinacea 38
enzyme 139
Epsom salts 128
essential fats 58
essential fatty acids 44
essential oils 15
estrogen 4
Europe 4

F

facial gel 111
FDA 141

female incontinence 53
Fenne 16
folic acid 24, 25, 139
fucus 68

G

geranium 117
ginkgo biloba 146
ginseng 141
glucosamine sulfate 84
Glycinemax 57
glycolic acid peels 121
growth hormone 75

H

hair loss 59
hawthorn 148
Herbs For fertility 30
Herbal fertility blend 31
hiatal hernia 43
high blood pressure 140, 148
HMO 137
honeysuckle 125
hormone depletion 59
hormone replacement therapy 47
hormones 15
hospital 136
hot tub 14
hydrochloric acid 43, 45

I

iodine 12
incontinence 53
iron 145

S

Seldane 47
selenium 145
serotonin 20
skating 85
skin care 120
skullcap 35
sleep 73
slimming tea blend 71
soap 105
soy 56, 57
spinning 151
strawberry 133
starvation gene 70
Synthroid 56

T

terpenes 147
textile arts 151
The Medical Letter 67
thyroxine 74
Tofu 56

U

U.S. Pharmacist 138
uterine 29

V

vegan 55
Vegetarian 55
Viacreme 52
violet 102, 131
vitamin A 35
vitamin C 56
Vitamin D 35
vitamin E 35
vitamins and minerals 30

W

watercress 71
weaving 151
weight control 65
wild yam root 44
wolfberry 145

Y

ylang ylang 103

Z

zinc gluconate 38

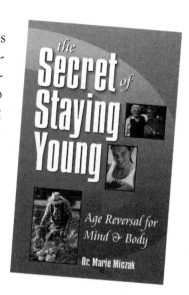

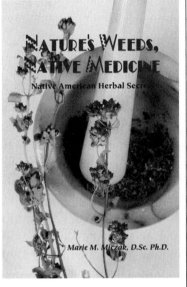

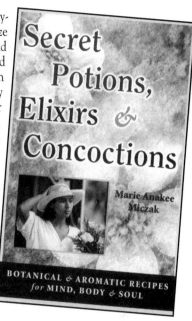